Textbook of Laser and Light Dermatology in the Asian Skin

Textbook of Laser and Light Dermatology in the Asian Skin

Editor

Yong-Kwang Tay

Changi General Hospital, Singapore

Co-Editor

Yuin-Chew Chan

Gleneagles Medical Centre, Singapore

World Scientific

NEW JERSEY · LONDON · SINGAPORE · BEIJING · SHANGHAI · HONG KONG · TAIPEI · CHENNAI

Published by

World Scientific Publishing Co. Pte. Ltd.
5 Toh Tuck Link, Singapore 596224
USA office: 27 Warren Street, Suite 401-402, Hackensack, NJ 07601
UK office: 57 Shelton Street, Covent Garden, London WC2H 9HE

Library of Congress Cataloging-in-Publication Data
Textbook of laser and light dermatology in the Asian skin / editor, Yong-Kwang Tay ; co-editor Yuin-Chew Chan.
p. ; cm.
Includes bibliographical references and index.
ISBN-13: 978-9814338868 (hardcover : alk. paper)
ISBN-10: 9814338869 (hardcover : alk. paper)
1. Skin--Diseases--Lasers in surgery. 2. Photodynamic therapy. 3. Asians--Surgery. I. Tay, Yong-Kwang. II. Chan, Yuin-Chew.
[DNLM: 1. Skin Diseases--therapy. 2. Asian Ancestry Group. 3. Cosmetic Techniques. 4. Laser Therapy--methods. 5. Photodynamic therapy--methods. WR 650]
RL120.P48T49 2011
617.4'770598--dc22

2011003151

British Library Cataloguing-in-Publication Data
A catalogue record for this book is available from the British Library.

Typeset by Stallion Press
Email: enquiries@stallionpress.com

Printed in Singapore.

Foreword

During the past decades our knowledge of laser surgery has undergone dramatic changes. New avenues of thinking have been opened and this has given patients with different types of lesions new treatment possibilities. Exciting improvements have been shown, but also the problems and side effects of treating pigmented Asian skin with lasers and light sources. Asian skin differs from Caucasian skin because of the higher amount of epidermal melanosomes and the higher level of melanin production.

Around 50% of the world population has darker skin types (Fitzpatrick skin types III–VI) and we need to learn more about how to treat them and how to avoid side effects like post-inflammatory hyperpigmentation. People travel and move around the world more than ever and all of us physicians need to have a higher understanding of the problems in treating darker skin types. This book will give you tips and tricks to avoid side effects and obtain better results.

This book is highly needed as, to my knowledge, there are not many books written regarding this subject. It reflects the tremendous progress in the field of laser dermatology. There is a growing number of skin lesions that are usually best treated with lasers or light sources. Research continues and new developments will allow us to improve patient care. This book will be of great value for dermatologists, plastic surgeons, pediatricians and general practitioners who will benefit from the many hours of clinical wisdom that have been distilled to produce it. The well-informed practicing dermatologist, using laser or light sources with skill and good judgment, can help solidify the image and substance of laser medicine and dermatology. I congratulate Dr Yong-Kwang Tay, FRCP and his co-authors and thank them for their devoted work.

To have a healthy-looking skin is a realistic dream for us all, no matter what skin type!

Agneta Troilius, MD, PhD
Head of the Laser & Vascular Anomaly Section at the
Department of Dermatology
Skånes University Hospital
Malmö, Sweden

Preface

Lasers have now been used in dermatology for over 40 years. The concept of selective photothermolysis transformed our understanding of laser-tissue interactions, and there has been an explosive interest in laser treatment for both skin diseases and aesthetic indications over the past decade or more.

For many years there has been awareness that the melanin content of skin can have profound implications on the outcome of laser treatment. Laser and light-based procedures in darker skin types have a significantly higher risk of complications, including scarring and pigmentary changes, compared to lighter skin types. It is essential that clinicians treating pigmented skin have a complete understanding of the implications of treatment of darker skin types.

There is thus a need for a textbook specifically addressing these issues in Asian skin. These needs are worldwide, as even in the northern hemisphere clinicians may need to treat a large immigrant population of Asian, Indian, and Hispanic descent with darker skin phototypes.

In this textbook, a series of clinicians from Singapore with extensive experience in treating Asian skin offer a comprehensive guide to treatment of this skin type. In addition to pigmentary differences, the manifestations of photoaging and cutaneous diseases can be different, as well as the responses to lasers in this population.

Effective treatment paradigms, as well as advice on complications and how to treat them, is provided for all areas of laser, intense pulsed light, and photodynamic treatment.

Chapters on laser-tissue interactions and laser safety introduce the subject and highlight many of the specific issues relating to treatment of Asian skin. *Textbook of Laser and Light Dermatology in the Asian Skin* is a most welcome and essential textbook. All clinicians treating darker skin types will benefit from reading this book, and they will certainly be better prepared to successfully treat patients with pigmented skin effectively and safely.

Sean Lanigan MD, FRCP, DCH
Consultant Dermatologist
Group Medical Director
Skin Clinic, Birmingham, UK

Acknowledgments

I am grateful to my colleagues who took time off, despite their busy schedules, to contribute chapters and make this textbook a reality. The authors are all experienced dermatologic laser surgeons who have given practical pearls of wisdom and tips to optimize outcomes when treating darker skin phototypes with lasers and light devices.

Special thanks to Dr Chan YC, my co-editor, Serene Lew, who provided expert secretarial assistance, and my international friends who generously shared their cases. I would also like to thank SingHealth Foundation, Changi General Hospital, Innomed and Medicare companies for their educational sponsorship.

This book is dedicated to my family: Wan Ching, Ern Wei, and Ern Ying for their continuous love, support, patience, and understanding in allowing me time to write and edit, and make everything worthwhile.

Finally, I hope that you, the reader, will find this book useful in your daily practice.

Yong-Kwang Tay, FRCP
Editor

List of Contributors

Por-Ang, *MBBS, MRCP (UK), FAMS (Dermatology)*
Consultant Dermatologist, Dermatology Associates,
Paragon Medical Centre, Singapore

Yuin-Chew Chan, *MBBS, MRCP (UK), FAMS (Dermatology)*
Consultant Dermatologist, Dermatology Associates,
Gleneagles Medical Centre, Singapore

Sze-Hon Chua, *MBBS, FRCP (Edin), FAMS (Dermatology)*
Senior Consultant Dermatologist,
Chief, Dermatological Surgery and Laser Unit,
National Skin Centre, Singapore

Melvin Ee, *MB ChB (UK), MRCP (UK), FAMS (Dermatology)*
Consultant Dermatologist,
Head, Skin Cancer Clinic, National Skin Centre
Singapore

Chee-Leok Goh, *MD, FRCP (Edin), FAMS (Dermatology)*
Senior Consultant Dermatologist, National Skin Centre, Singapore
Clinical Professor, National University of Singapore
Adjunct Professor, Duke-NUS Graduate Medical School

Colin Kwok, *MBBS, FRCP (Edin), FAMS (Dermatology)*
Senior Consultant Dermatologist,
Department of Dermatology,
Changi General Hospital, Singapore

Su-Ping Lim, **Regina**, *MBBCh (UK), MRCP (UK), FAMS (Dermatology)*
Consultant Dermatologist,
Department of Dermatology,
Changi General Hospital, Singapore

Joyce Teng-Ee Lim, *MBBS (MAL), FRCP (Ire), FAMS (Dermatology)*
Consultant Dermatologist,
Joyce Lim Skin and Laser Clinic,
Paragon Medical Centre, Singapore

Eileen Tan, *MRCP (UK), M.Med (Int Med), FAMS (Dermatology)*
Consultant Dermatologist,
Eileen Tan Skin, Laser and Hair Transplant Clinic,
Mount Elizabeth Medical Centre, Singapore

Yong-Kwang Tay, *FRCP (Lond), FRCP (Ire), FAMS (Dermatology)*
Chief and Senior Consultant,
Department of Dermatology
Changi General Hospital, Singapore

Colin Thiam-Seng Theng, *MBBS, MRCP (UK), FAMS (Dermatology)*
Consultant Dermatologist,
Chief, Psoriasis and Phototherapy Unit,
National Skin Centre, Singapore

Su-Ni Wong, *MRCP (UK), M.Med (Int Med), FAMS (Dermatology)*
Consultant Dermatologist,
Dr SN Wong Skin, Hair, Nails & Lasers Specialist Clinic,
Mount Elizabeth Medical Centre, Singapore

Contents

Chapter 1

Laser and Light-Tissue Interactions

Melvin Ee*

Introduction

Albert Einstein first conceptualized the idea of stimulated emission in 1917. At that time, few realized the potential of this concept. It was not till the 1950s that MASER (Microwave Amplification by Stimulated Emission of Radiation) was discovered that the possibility of inducing stimulated emission in the visible light region of the electromagnetic spectrum was investigated.[1] In 1960, Maiman introduced the first functional laser consisting of a flashlamp pump device incorporating a ruby crystal that produced laser light at a wavelength of 694 nm.[2]

Development of other lasers followed quickly: neodymium:yttrium-aluminum-garnet (Nd:YAG, 1961), argon (1962), carbon dioxide (CO_2) (1964) and dye laser (1966) were the first few lasers manufactured. In 1983, a fundamental breakthrough in the understanding of laser/light interactions with the skin was published as the "Theory of Selective Photothermolysis."[3] This allowed the targeting of specific constituents of the skin without damaging the surrounding tissues. Over time, this translated clinically into the development of more sophisticated laser devices for the treatment of a variety of medical conditions.

Laser

LASER is an acronym for Light Amplification by Stimulated Emission of Radiation. Laser systems (Fig. 1.1) comprise basically four essential components. These include:

1. Laser Pumping System

The unit here provides energy to the laser system. Although the energy sources are usually light and electric current, chemical and even nuclear energy may be used. The energy is transferred into the gain medium exciting the atoms. These become unstable and will release their energy in the form of photons, allowing excited higher orbit electrons to move back to their ground state. This process is known as spontaneous emission. Subsequently, "population inversion" is said to have occurred if more than half of the atoms within the gain medium are in an excited state.

2. Optical Cavity

This is considered the heart of the laser machine. It consists of a highly reflective chamber flanked by a fully reflective mirror and a partially reflective mirror encasing the gain medium. Lasers are named after their respective mediums and they may be semiconductors or exist in a gaseous (e.g. carbon dioxide, excimer), solid (e.g. ruby, alexandrite, neodymium: yttrium-aluminum-garnet, erbium:yttrium-aluminum-garnet), or liquid state (e.g. dye). Semiconductors are electronic devices which have the capability of generating high power with little energy.

*Consultant Dermatologist, Head, Skin Cancer Clinic, National Skin Centre, Singapore.

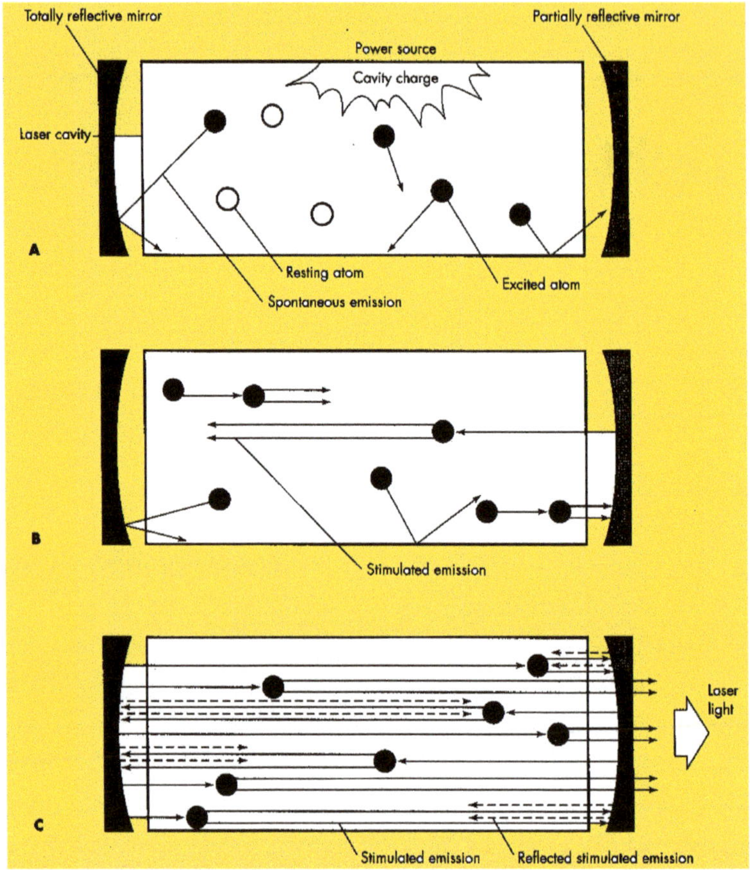

Figure 1.1.

The essential components of a laser system.

The photon emitted is of a specific wavelength and phase and is determined by the specific gain medium. Within the optical cavity, these photons are reflected back and forth between the mirrors and in their course excite other atoms, which emit exponentially more photons of the same wavelength and phase. This cascade effect results in the process of stimulated emission.

While the fully reflective mirror reflects all photons, the partially reflective mirror allows some photons through into the delivery system.

3. Delivery System

The laser emitted from the partially reflective mirror now enters a delivery system, which may consist of fibreoptic cables (e.g. VBeam^{TM}, Candela) or a series of reflective mirrors based within the articulated arms (e.g. Medlite^{TM}, QS Nd:YAG, Con Bio). The latter may be considered a more robust and sturdier system. Though the fiberoptic delivery system may be light and maneuverable, they have a fundamental limit in the intensity of the light that it can transmit in the fiber. It is unable to deliver high intensity energies as the optical nonlinearities induced within it can prevent laser operation and/or lead to the material destruction of the fiber.

4. Handpiece

The delivery system terminates in the handpiece, which may emit the laser as a collimated beam or focused beam with the aid of lenses.

Unlike standard light sources, laser exhibits three unique characteristics. These are:

1. Monochromacity

When an excited and unstable atom releases a photon of energy, electrons will revert back to their stable original orbit. The photons emitted are identical and the light emission contains only one wavelength, which is determined by the laser medium.

2. Coherence

Light can be envisaged as a sine wave. In this context, it travels in phase, both spatially and temporally. Each photon moves in step with one another with military precision.

3. Focused

Laser light waves run parallel. As such, the diameter of the beam produced is fixed. It is also of high intensity and able to travel distances with negligible loss of intensity. Furthermore, this parallel beam can be focused to very small spot sizes using a suitable lens. This is widely used in carbon dioxide laser systems which employs focused beams for "bloodless" excisions while using the parallel beams for resurfacing purposes.

Laser Pulse Characteristics

Lasers may be further classified based on pulse characteristics, i.e. they may be continuous, pulsed or Q-switched.

Continuous wave lasers (Fig. 1.2) are usually seen in carbon dioxide and argon lasers. The laser emitted

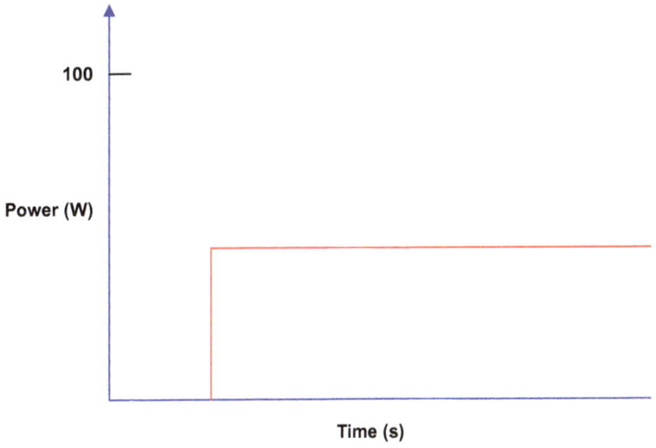

Figure 1.2.

Continuous wave laser.

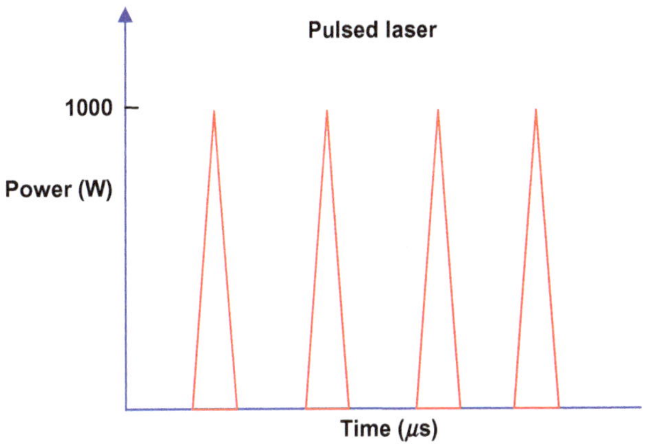

Figure 1.3.

Pulsed lasers produce short individual pulses of high peak power.

is without interruption (continuously) and of low power.

This output remains constant, whereas in a pulsed mode (Fig. 1.3), the laser beam is emitted in a train of narrow, higher peak power pulses with predetermined on- and off time cycles even though the laser switch is depressed. The higher peak power is achieved through pulsing the laser over a shorter period of time. With higher peak powers, tissue incision capability is enhanced. At the same time, with a shorter laser activation time, collateral tissue has more time to cool between pulses, translating to reduced probab-ility of thermal damage. If the laser is able to generate a succession of pulses at a high enough repetition rate to appear continuous, it may be labeled as quasicontinuous.

Modification to the above results in superpulsing which generates an even higher peak power. Examples of pulsed lasers are pulsed dye laser and ultrapulsed CO_2 laser.

Even higher peak energies can be achieved if the pulse duration is shortened (nanosecond range). This technique is utilized in Q-switched lasers. "Q" refers to the quality factor of the laser cavity and represents the rate of discharge of energy. Q-switching refers to an electromagnetic or chemical switch within the laser cavity that allows the release of all the energy in one brief powerful pulse (Fig. 1.4). This is achieved through inclusion of some type of variable attenuator inside the laser's optical cavity. When the attenuator is functioning, light which leaves the gain medium does not return, and lasing cannot begin. Initially, the laser medium is pumped while the Q-switch is set to prevent feedback of light into the gain medium. This produces a population inversion, but laser operation cannot yet occur since there is no feedback from the cavity. The amount of energy stored in the gain medium increases as the medium is pumped. After a certain time the stored energy will reach a maximum level. At this point, the Q-switch device is quickly changed, allowing feedback and the process of optical amplification by stimulated emission to begin. Because of the large amount of energy already stored in the gain medium, the intensity of light in the laser cavity builds up very quickly; this also causes the energy stored in the medium to be depleted almost as quickly. The net result is a short pulse of light output from the laser, with very high peak intensity.

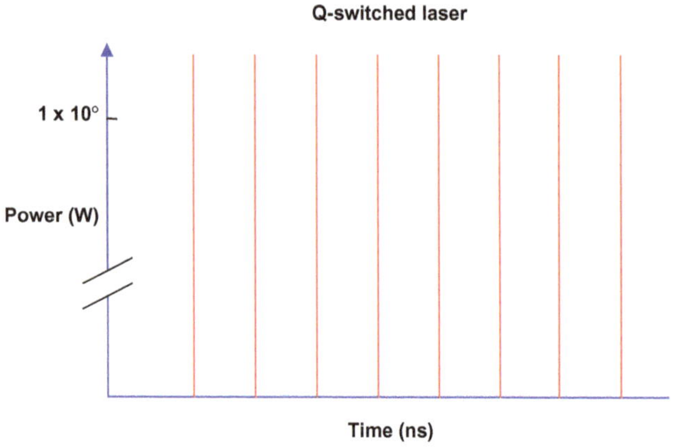

Figure 1.4.

Q-switched lasers produce pulses of very short duration and extremely high power.

Tissue Optics and Lights

Light may be reflected from or may enter the skin when it strikes the air–skin interface. The minority (approximately 4%) of the incident light is reflected. This occurs as a result of the difference between the refractive index of air and skin. This reflectance of light is determined by the refractive indices of the media, the angles that the incident, reflected and refracted rays make to the interface and the plane of polarization. The epidermis is responsible for most of the reflection from the skin.

The remaining light upon entering the skin may be absorbed, scattered or transmitted. Within the skin, absorption is one of the dominant processes over the ultraviolet (UV) and mid-infrared spectra. The relationship of the absorption of light to the properties of the material through which the light is traveling is best described by Beer's law. It states that the optical absorbance of a chromophore in a homogenous medium varies linearly with the medium path length, the chromophore concentration and absorption affinity. When light is absorbed, it gives up its photon to a target molecule termed a chromophore. The photon will cease to exist and this quantum of energy transferred excites the chromophore. Without light absorption, there can be no effect on the tissue. In the skin, the three main primary chromophores are melanin, water and hemoglobin. Each of these exhibits its particular band of absorption at certain wavelengths (Fig. 1.5). Melanin, which is predominantly found in the epidermis and hair follicles, may also be found in the

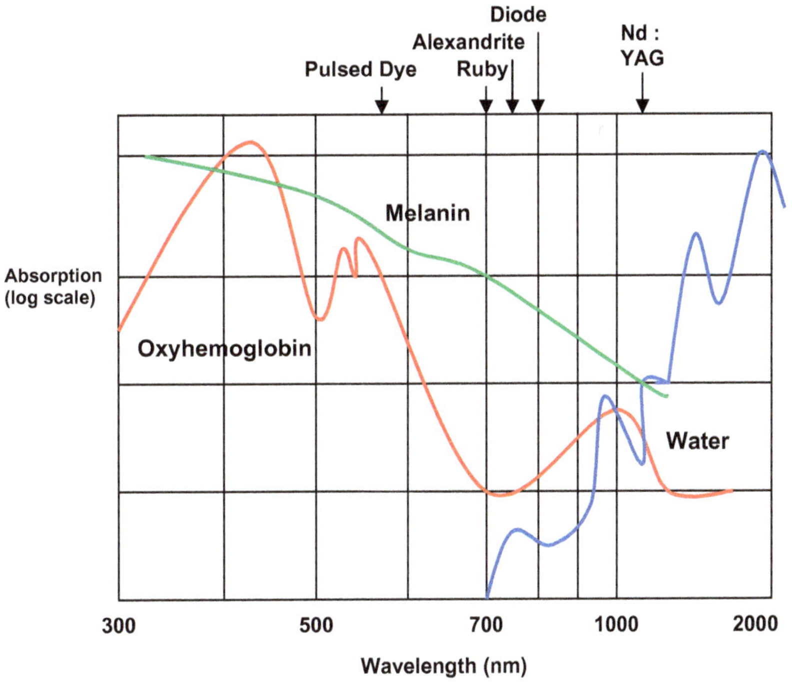

Figure 1.5.

Absorption spectrum of major chromophores in the skin.

dermis. As its main function is to protect against the detrimental effects of sunlight, its absorption spectrum include mainly ultraviolet and visible light. Water, the main component of collagen, absorbs best beyond the near infrared spectra. Hemoglobin, on the other hand, exhibits peak absorption in the UVA, blue (400 nm), green (541 nm) and yellow (577 nm) wavelengths. With this in mind, the properties of light can be manipulated in terms of its wavelength, pulse duration and energy (fluence) such that a particular chromophore is preferentially targeted, absorbing the light energy and is destroyed while other chromophores are left intact.

Scattering, the other dominant process within the skin, occurs when the incident light is forced to deviate from a straight trajectory by one or more localized non-uniformities in the medium through which they pass. In the skin, collagen fibrils causes most of the scattering. Clinically this is an important concept as scattering reduces the available fluence for absorption and as such potentially decreases the desired effect on the targeted chromophore. The effect of scattering proportionately decreases with increasing wavelengths. This, on the other hand, makes it an ideal modality to reach deeper target tissues based within the deeper dermis, e.g. hair follicles or dermal melanin. In practice, due to lower scattering, a longer wavelength, e.g. 1064 nm laser, will not only be able to penetrate to the level of the deep dermis, to the targeted hair or melanin, but there is also limited absorption by other endogenous chromophores at this wavelength.

The residual light, which has not been absorbed or scattered in the tissue, will be transmitted into the subcutaneous tissues. These are mainly beyond the 700 nm spectra.

Light Tissue Interactions

Various parameters (Table 1.1) e.g. wavelength, fluence, power, spot size, pulse duration and cooling

Table 1.1.

Common Laser Terminology

Term	What it Means	Units
Chromophore	Substance that absorbs light	NA
Wavelength	The distance between one peak or crest of a wave of light and the next corresponding peak or crest.	nanometers (nm)
Pulse Duration/ width	The length of time that the laser is exposed to the skin	nanoseconds (ns) milliseconds (ms)
Fluence	The amount of energy delivered to a unit square area	J/cm^2
Power	The rate at which energy is delivered	W
Spot size	The diameter of the laser upon skin impact	millimeters (mm)

Table 1.2.

Selective Photothermolysis Targets

Chromophore	TRT	Pulsewidth	Laser
Tattoo/pigment	ns	ns	Q-switched
Blood vessel, Telangiectasia	ms	ms	Pulsed dye
Venule	sec (s)	ms	Long pulsed
Hair follicle	ms	ms	Long pulsed

method affect laser tissue interactions. Depending on these qualities, the reaction of the tissue to light/laser irradiation is as follows:

1. Photothermolytic Reactions

Laser/light tissue interactions invariably produce heat which can denature various cells, e.g. melanocytes, keratinocytes or essential structures, e.g. collagen and blood vessels which make up the skin. Each component within the skin has a threshold for heat injury before it denatures. As such, precise placement of the heat generated by laser/light interactions both spatially and sequentially may preferentially cause damage to the target tissue and at the same time preserve surrounding tissues.

Once a laser impacts the skin, it is absorbed by the tissue producing heat. Thermal relaxation time (TRT) is the time required for the targeted heated tissue to lose half its heat. Therefore the key to successful laser treatment is to affect a thermal effect in the target tissue quickly and cause damage to it before the heat is conducted to the surrounding tissue.

In other words, if we carefully select the laser/light wavelength, with an appropriate fluence and a pulse duration equal or less that the TRT of the target, focal selective destruction of the target occurs with little or no destruction to surrounding tissue (Table 1.2). If the conditions are met, the heat generated should reside within the target until it is damaged without heat dis-spitating to the surrounding tissue. As a result this will only require minimum light/laser deposition and provide selective damage. This forms the basic concept of "selective photothermolysis."

Chromophores may also be used as subsurface heat sources to denature nearby tissue targets. This is known as the "extended theory of selective photothermolysis."[4] This is best illustrated in the scenarios involving hair removal and the treatment of telangiectasias. In hair removal, the chromophore is the melanin in the hair shaft while the target structures like the stem cells within the bulge area have little melanin content. If a longer pulse width is utilized, the melanin laden hairshaft is heated up and significant heat diffusion damages the target stem cells. By the same reasoning, in the treatment of telangiectasias, the laser targets hemoglobin, heats it up and heat then diffuses to the blood vessel wall, coagulating it.[5]

2. Photochemical/Photodynamic Reactions

The process usually involves the administration of either a topical or systemic photosensitizer that is subsequently activated by a light or laser source to destroy targeted tissues. With an appropriate light source (e.g. laser, noncoherent light or light emitting diodes), the photosensitizer is excited and subsequently transfers its energy to generate reactive oxygen species within the targeted tissues. The reactive oxygen species causes selective tumor destruction. For example, the tumor selectivity of photodynamic therapy in the treatment of superficial non-melanoma skin cancer is based on the application of the agent (5-aminolevulinic acid) to the tumor (Bowen's disease or superficial basal cell carcinoma) for 3–4 hours, and then irradiated with red light. The photochemical reaction takes place during illumination with selective destruction and necrosis of the tumor cells.

3. Photomechanical Reactions

These are induced mainly by high power, short pulse lasers.[6] The generation of laser-induced stress waves can disrupt tissue, kill cells, decrease cell viability and increase the permeability of the plasma membrane.[7] Additionally, it may cause erythrocyte vaporization and mechanical vessel rupture with hemorrhage.

4. Photostimulatory Reactions

Experimentally, it has been shown that low energy level laser may be beneficial for wound healing.[8–10] Although the results suggest possible mechanisms by which the wavelength may potentially influence the cellular responses of injured cells,[11] more work has to be done before the concept can be translated into clinical practice.

Tissue Cooling

Tissue cooling is of paramount importance and has been incorporated into many laser systems. During laser treatment of vascular lesions and hair removal, it is inevitable that epidermal melanin may become an undesired target chromophore. Although this may not be an issue in fairer skin individuals, pigmented skin types may suffer pigmentary side effects or blistering with scar formation. The use of tissue cooling minimizes this risk of epidermal heat accumulation and damage.

Techniques employed to cool tissue vary between different laser manufacturers. In essence, cooling methods involve either the convection or conduction of heat through the surface of the skin. To enhance this process, a gradient of cooler temperature is created on the surface of the skin through one or more of the following processes.[12]

1. Cold Air Convection

Ambient room air is cooled down to –30°C using a closed loop cooling circuit before targeting it at the area of laser treatment. It may also minimize pain during laser treatments.

2. Contact Cooling

The cooling agent may include chilled liquid between transparent plates through which the laser fires through, which abuts the skin. Sapphire is usually used as it is a much better conductor than glass and its thermal conductivity approaches that of metals. Others may incorporate a chilled moving solid, e.g. copper, as means of heat extraction. These are specially chosen for their high thermal conductivity. Cold gel acts via passive contact cooling. For maximal heat transfer to occur, the contact between skin and the cooling agent must be excellent. To achieve this, firm pressure of the device coupled with gel can be applied together.

3. Dynamic Cryogen Cooling

Here, targeted bursts of cryogen impacts on the skin, allowing evaporative cooling to take place milliseconds before the laser pulse. This method is able to achieve cooling of the tissue up to a depth and temperature of 1 mm and −20°C, respectively.

Cooling may also be divided into three arbitrary phases: pre-cooling, parallel cooling and post-cooling which refers to cooling before, during and after laser exposure.[12] In Q-switched systems, as the pulse duration is very short (nanoseconds), it is difficult to sufficiently cool the skin and pre-cooling is appropriate, providing the epidermal protection. Parallel cooling is more suitable for laser systems with longer pulse durations. Post-cooling may further protect the epidermis as well as reduce discomfort, swelling and erythema.

With cooling, we can expect increased comfort as well as reduced risk of heat accumulation, especially during treatments at higher energy fluence. This in turn can translate to a better clinical outcome. It has been said that cooling will also allow the treatment of darker skin types. This may be true if cooling is used judiciously. Excessive cooling, on the other hand, may cause cryogen-induced injury.

Cryogen-induced injury is more commonly reported in pigmented skin. Post-inflammatory hyperpigmentation due to cold air convection techniques has been reported.[13] A split face study involving 21 patients undergoing Q-switched Nd:YAG laser treatments for Hori's nevus showed that the cooled sides were significantly more likely to become hyperpigmented after laser irradiation as compared with the uncooled sides. Cryogen-induced arcuate shaped hyperpigmentation has also been reported in dynamic cooling devices.[14]

Conclusion

A good understanding of laser/light-skin interactions will enable one to choose an appropriate device and to optimize laser parameters so as to achieve the desired clinical end point resulting in more effective and safer laser/light treatments in all skin phototypes.

References

1. Townes CH. (1962) Optical masers and their possible applications to biology. *Biophys J* **2**: 325–329.
2. Maiman TH. (1966) Biomedical lasers evolve toward clinical applications. *Hosp Manage* **101**: 39–41.
3. Anderson RR, Parrish JA. (1983) Selective photothermolysis: precise microsurgery by selective absorption of pulsed radiation. *Science* **220**: 524–527.
4. Altshuler GB, Anderson RR, Manstein D, *et al.* (2001) Extended theory of selective photothermolysis. *Lasers Surg Med* **29**: 416–432.
5. Garden JM, Tan OT, Kerschmann R, *et al.* (1986) Effect of dye laser pulse duration on selective cutaneous vascular injury. *J Invest Dermatol* **87**: 653–657.
6. Watanabe S, Flotte TJ, McAuliffe DJ, *et al.* (1988) Putative photoacoustic damage in skin induced by pulsed ArF excimer laser. *J Invest Dermatol* **90**: 761–766.
7. Doukas AG, Flotte TJ. (1996) Physical characteristics and biological effects of laser-induced stress waves. *Ultrasound Med Biol* **22**: 151–164.
8. Reddy GK. (2004) Photobiological basis and clinical role of low-intensity lasers in biology and medicine. *J Clin Laser Med Surg* **22**: 141–150.
9. Posten W, Wrone DA, Dover JS, *et al.* (2005) Low-level laser therapy for wound healing: mechanism and efficacy. *Dermatol Surg* **31**: 334–340.
10. Skopin MD, Molitor SC. (2009) Effects of near-infrared laser exposure in a cellular model of wound healing. *Photodermatol Photoimmunol Photomed* **25**: 75–80.
11. Evans DH, Abrahamse H. (2008) Efficacy of three different laser wavelengths for in vitro wound healing. *Photodermatol Photoimmunol Photomed* **24**: 199–210.
12. Zenzie HH, Altshuler GB, Smirnov MZ, *et al.* (2000) Evaluation of cooling methods for laser dermatology. *Lasers Surg Med* **26**: 130–144.
13. Manuskiatti W, Eimpunth S, Wanitphakdeedecha R. (2007) Effect of cold air cooling on the incidence of postinflammatory hyperpigmentation after Q-switched Nd:YAG laser treatment of acquired bilateral nevus of Ota like macules. *Arch Dermatol* **143**: 1139–1143.
14. Lee SJ, Park SG, Kang JM, *et al.* (2008) Cryogen-induced arcuate shaped hyperpigmentation by dynamic cooling device. *J Eur Acad Dermatol Venereol* **22**: 883–884.

Chapter 2

Laser Safety

Su-Ni Wong*

Introduction

The safe use of lasers entails knowledge of the laser characteristics (Table 2.1), laser-tissue interactions, and optimal treatment parameters for various skin types, as well as provision of a safe environment for both the patient and the operator, with adequate protection against laser-related hazards. These would vary from one laser machine to another, and guidance should be sought from the manufacturer or distributor when purchasing the laser or setting up the laser room.

Laser safety encompasses several areas:[1]

1. Adequate training
2. Medical surveillance
3. Laser Hazards Analysis
4. Provision of safe environment
5. Personal protective equipment

Adequate Training

Doctors should ensure that they have received adequate training, including hands-on training, and accreditation in the use of the laser equipment before offering it as a service to their patients.[2,3] Training courses, encompassing laser physics, laser safety, clinical indications, laser techniques, pre- and post-operative care, laser complications, and hands-on training, are usually offered by professional societies such as the American Society for Laser Medicine and Surgery, the American Academy of Dermatology, and the Dermatological Society of Singapore.[4] Medical lasers used in dermatology are mostly Class 3 lasers, and emit non-ionizing radiation. As such, they are regulated in Singapore under the Radiation Protection Act 2007, and a separate license is required for owning and operating each laser.[5] Licensing requirements, including pre-licensing training or tests, vary from country to country and advice should be sought from the relevant authorities.

In certain countries, e.g. Singapore, laser procedures are performed only by the licensed doctor and not by nursing or non-medical staff. In some countries, light-based treatments and nonablative esthetic laser procedures may be delegated to responsible and trained medical personnel under the direct supervision of a trained and certified doctor.[6] There should be written and precise protocols with respect to the specific laser and specific site treated, and the supervising doctor should be available immediately and able to respond quickly should any untoward events occur.[6] The supervising doctor is ultimately responsible for the safety and outcome of the laser procedure.

Doctors performing laser procedures should familiarize themselves with the early recognition, prevention, and management of post-laser complications such as blisters, burns, scarring, and postinflammatory dyspigmentation.

A laser safety officer should be appointed (usually the doctor or the nursing officer in charge of the surgical suites) to oversee all aspects of laser safety,

*Dr. SN Wong Skin, Hair, Nails & Lasers Specialist Clinic, Mt Elizabeth Medical Centre, Singapore. Visiting Consultant, National Skin Centre, Singapore.

Table 2.1.

Common Lasers and their Wavelengths

Laser Type	Examples	Wavelength	Target Chromophore
Carbon dioxide (CO_2)	Sharplan™ Ultrapulse™ SmartXide DOT™ Mixto SX™ Fraxel Re:pair™ Deep FX™	10,600 nm	Water
Erbium:YAG	Sciton Profile Contour™	2940 nm	Water
Erbium-doped fibre	Fraxel Re:store™	1550 nm	Water
Erbium-Glass	Lux1540 Fractional™ Mosaic™	1540 nm	Water
Q-switched Nd:YAG	Medlite™	1064 nm 532 nm (frequency-doubled)	Melanin Epidermal melanin
Long pulsed Nd:YAG	CoolGlide™ Sciton Profile Clearscan™ Gentle-YAG™	1064 nm	Melanin, hemoglobin
Diode	SmoothBeam™ ELOS e-Laser™	1450 nm 900 nm	Water Hemoglobin, melanin
Pulsed dye	V-Beam™	585, 595 nm	Hemoglobin, melanin

including ensuring that all staff assisting in laser procedures are trained in laser safety and proper handling of laser equipment and that all safety policies and procedures are followed, with regular maintenance and servicing of laser equipment.[7] It is helpful to designate a laser room nurse to be in charge of day-to-day setting up and maintenance of the laser equipment.

Medical Surveillance

A baseline eye examination is usually required before a laser license is issued for the use of Class 3 lasers (Fig. 2.1). Care should be taken to document pre-existing eye problems, and conditions that lower the threshold for biological effects on the cornea, lens, and retina should be elicited. A baseline skin examination is required for those with a history of photosensitivity or working with ultraviolet lasers. High-intensity, visible light (e.g. intense pulsed light) is also capable of increasing the risk of eye damage, and eye examination should be offered to those working with these devices to monitor for adverse effects.

Table 2.2.

Biological Effects of Light of Different Wavelengths

Photobiological Spectrum	Effect on Eye	Effect on Skin
Ultraviolet B (280–315 nm)	Photokeratitis	Skin burn Accelerated skin aging Increased pigmentation
Ultraviolet A (315–400 nm)	Photochemical cataract	Pigment darkening Skin burn
Visible (400–780 nm)	Photochemical and thermal retinal injury	Photosensitive reactions
Infrared A (780–1400 nm)	Cataract, retinal burn	Skin burn
Infrared B (1400–3000 nm)	Corneal burn Aqueous flare Cataract	Skin burn
Infrared C (3000–10,000 nm)	Corneal burn	Skin burn

MEDICAL CERTIFICATE FOR LASER OPERATORS

HISTORY	
	Family:
	Medical:
	Occupational:
CLINICAL & SPECIAL INVESTIGATION (SATISFACTORY/UNSATISFACTORY) §	
	Dermatological:
	Others:
OPHTHALMOLOGICAL EXAMINATION (SATISFACTORY/UNSATISFACTORY) §	
	Date of Examination:
	Medical History of Eyes:
	Colour Vision:
	Visual Acuity Far: Near:
	Amsler Grid:
	Manifest Refraction:
	External Ocular Examination:
	Examination of the Ocular Fundus with an ophthalmoscope:
	Other Examinations:
	Optional: Examination by slit lamp: Tonometry:

Figure 2.1.

Example of a baseline medical examination required for laser users. (*Source*: National Environmental Agency, Singapore.)

Photograph of Posterior: Pole of the Fundus:
STATEMENT
This is to certify that: Dr/Mr/Ms/Mdm: ______ NRIC No.: ______ Employed by: ______ has undergone a medical examination by me and I am of the opinion that he/she§ is fit/unfit§ to engaged in laser work. In addition, I have the following comments to make: ______ ______ ______ Date ______ Signature of Medical Practitioner ______ Address of Hospital/Clinic ______ Name of Medical Practitioner

§ Delete as applicable.

Figure 2.1. ***(Continued)***

Laser Hazards

Laser hazards can be broadly divided into beam-related hazards and non-beam hazards.[1]

Beam-related hazards relate to the effects of the laser beam on the eye and skin. Acute exposure of the eye to lasers of certain wavelengths (e.g. 1064 nm Nd:YAG and 10,600 nm CO_2 laser) and power can cause corneal[8–10] retinal burns,[11,12] or macular injury.[13,14] Chronic exposure to excessive levels of laser light in the ultraviolet, visible, or infrared range may cause corneal opacities, cataracts, or retinal injury.[15] High-power laser beams may cause skin burns, ignite flammable materials, and heat materials that release hazardous fumes, gases, or debris. Increased risk of carcinogenesis, although not yet clinically proven, is an issue to consider with use of ultraviolet and near-ultraviolet wavelengths (e.g. 308 nm XeCl Excimer laser).[16,17]

Non-beam hazards include electrical hazards, chemical hazards, fire hazards, and health hazards from inhalation of the laser plume generated while using ablative lasers, e.g. CO_2 or erbium:YAG lasers.[18,19] Some lasers require hazardous or toxic substances to operate (e.g. pulsed dye, excimer lasers). Fire hazard arises when all three elements of the fire triad are present: fuel, oxidizer, and ignition.[20] The solvents used in dye lasers are flammable, as are alcohol-based disinfectants and antiseptics.[21,22] Oxygen provided during general anesthesia increases the risk.[23] High-voltage pulse or flash lamps, or diathermy, may cause ignition. Flammable materials may be ignited by direct beams or reflections from mirror-like surfaces.

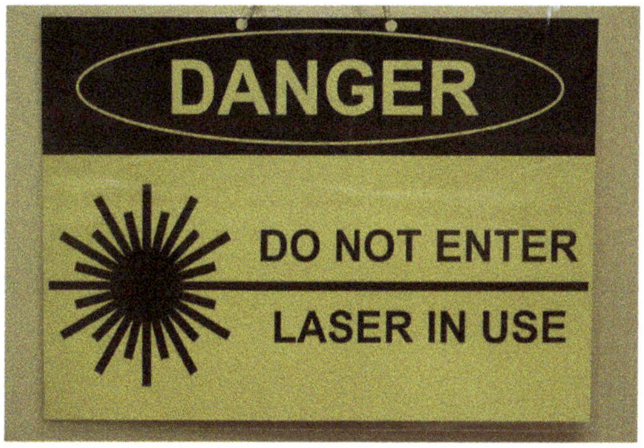

Figure 2.2.

Laser warning sign prominently displayed on the door when the laser is in use.

Provision of Safe Environment

After the potential hazards have been identified, the doctor in charge has to ensure that these hazards are minimized by careful construction and design of the laser room, implementation of standard operating protocols for each laser used, regular laser servicing and maintenance, and consistent use of personal protective equipment by all laser room staff and patients.

A laser room should be fully enclosed with floor-to-ceiling walls, with limited access when a laser procedure is underway. Access to the area during a laser procedure should require the permission of the laser operator. The windows should be covered with curtains, blinds, or other nonreflective material, and there should not be reflective surfaces such as mirrors within the room.[24] A fire extinguisher should be available and staff should be trained to use it. Power points should be appropriate for the requirements of the laser machine, and should not be overloaded by the use of multiple adapters. The door should be made of an opaque and nonreflective material. A laser warning sign (Fig. 2.2) and a warning light should be prominently displayed outside the door while laser procedures are performed.[7]

A smoke evacuator is essential when ablative lasers (e.g. CO_2 laser) are used, to reduce the risk of transmission of viral infections (from viral particles present in the laser plume) as well as upper respiratory tract irritation. Surgical masks should be worn by both the laser operator and assistant during ablative laser procedures. Human papilloma virus-DNA has been detected in laser as well as diathermy plume generated during excision of papillomas and condylomas.[25,26] A bovine inoculation study demonstrated that the inoculation of CO_2 laser plume (extracted during CO_2 laser excision of bovine cutaneous fibropapillomas) into the skin of calves resulted in tumor growth at the inoculated sites of the same papilloma virus type as that present in the laser plume.[27] Laryngeal papillomatosis has also been recognized as an occupational hazard in laser surgeons and operating room nurses, likely contracted via inhalation of the laser plume, particularly when performing CO_2 laser excision of anogenital warts.[28,29] Surgical plumes, like other smoke plumes, contain carbon monoxide, polyaromatic hydrocarbons, and a variety of toxic gases. Hence, they can produce upper respiratory tract irritation, and have *in vitro* mutagenic potential.[30]

Smoke evacuators may be handheld, requiring an assistant to hold the flexible hose, or stand-alone, with rigid but movable arms (Fig. 2.3). The evacuator should have a high efficiency particulate air filter (HEPA) to filter out particulate matter. The capture velocity should be about 100–150 feet per minute at the inlet nozzle, which should be held about 5 cm above the operation site for effective removal of plume.[24]

Protocols on safe laser use should be readily available in each laser room. Laser machines often come with a key lock — only authorized users should be

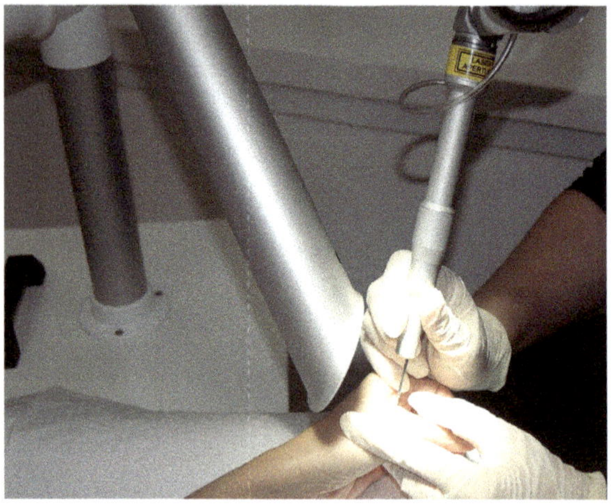

Figure 2.3.

A smoke evacuator with rigid but movable arms is very useful for ablative laser and diathermy procedures, leaving the assistant's hands free to assist in other ways. The nozzle should be at most 5 cm away from the area being lasered, and the plume visibly drawn into the tube.

allowed access to the key. The laser machine should be on standby mode when not in direct use. It should be turned off and unplugged after use, with the key removed and kept in a secure place.

Personal Protective Equipment

Eye Protection

Goggles of sufficient optical density intended to protect from the specific laser wavelength are to be used by all persons in the laser room. It is the responsibility of the laser operator to ensure that everyone in the room is protected before starting the laser procedure (Fig. 2.4).

It is important to note that goggles designed for protection at one wavelength may offer little or no protection against another wavelength.[31] The optical density and wavelengths for which protection is offered should be clearly labeled on the eye wear. To avoid confusion, it is advisable to keep the appropriate goggles for the specific laser machine on the machine itself. The patient is given either the same

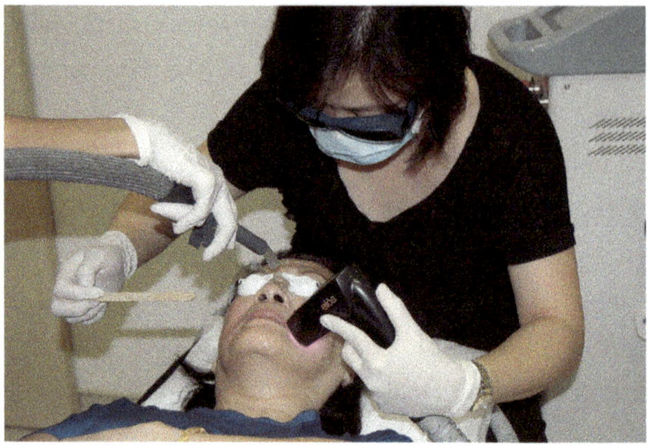

Figure 2.4.

Laser-opaque external eye shield is used for the patient and protective goggles for the laser operator and assistant.

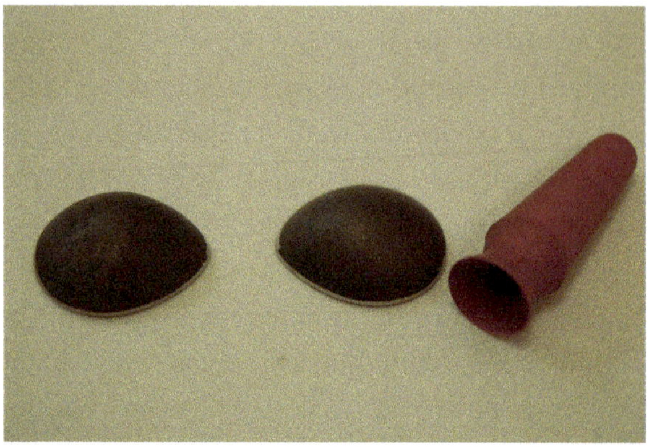

Figure 2.5.

Autoclavable eye shields recommended for Nd:YAG and ablative laser procedures performed near the eyes. These are inserted using the rubber lens holder after instillation of anesthetic eye drops.

goggles or a laser-opaque shield. For procedures around the eyes or on the eyelids, internal eye shields made of laser-opaque material are to be used (Fig. 2.5). For most lasers, metal eye shields are the most appropriate. The eye wear should be inspected periodically for pitting and cracking of the lenses, and for mechanical integrity in the frame.

Reflective jewelry should be removed before the laser procedure. Lasers should not be directed at the eye or at another person.

Although intense pulsed light (IPL) is not a laser, eye protection should also be worn during IPL procedures, as intense visible light is also capable of producing light-induced retinal damage (LIRD), with effects similar to but more aggressive than age-related macular degeneration (AMD).[32]

Skin Protection

The untreated skin may be protected through use of clothing or drapes to cover normally exposed skin areas. Drapes or gauze moistened with water confer good protection for the surrounding skin while performing CO_2 laser ablation or during general anesthesia in a child undergoing pulsed dye laser treatments to prevent fire hazards. Care should be taken to drape or avoid hairlines that may have hairspray or other flammable solutions dried in the hairline. Use of non-flammable petrolatum over hair-bearing areas is also helpful to reduce the risk of laser fire.

Conclusion

Laser safety involves both engineering as well as behavioral aspects. Regardless of how well designed the laser facilities are, and how well equipped with protective features and personal protective gear, there is no substitute for common sense and adherence to good safety practices. Hazards can be significantly reduced or eliminated with adherence to well-communicated safety protocols. It is imperative that the operating physician take the lead in ensuring that these protocols are followed.

References

1. ANSI Z136.3–2005. Standard for the safe use of lasers in health care facilities. American National Standards Institute 2005.
2. Alam M. (2007) Who is qualified to perform laser surgery and in what setting? *Semin Plast Surg* **21**: 193–200.
3. Drake LA, Ceilley RI, Cornelison RL, *et al.* (1995) Standards of training for physicians for the use of lasers in Medicine and Surgery, American Society for Laser Medicine and Surgery, Inc. *J Am Acad Dermatol* **33**: 265–270.
4. Dermatological Society of Singapore (2010). Retrieved 17 April 2010, from http://www.dermatology.org.sg/events.htm.
5. National Environmental Agency, Singapore, 2010. Retrieved 17 April 2010, from http://app2.nea.gov.sg/licenses.aspx#radiation.
6. Board of Directors, American Society of Laser Medicine and Surgery. (1999) ASLMS principles for non-physician laser use. *American Society of Laser Medicine and Surgery*, Apr 15.
7. Absten G. (2006) Laser safety operational guidelines — office dermatology procedures: Policies and procedures. Retrieved on 17 April 2010, from http://www.lasertraining.org/.../Laser%20Policies%20-%20Office%20Dermatology-Aesthetic%20Sample%20Policies%20Feb06.doc.
8. Widder RA, Severin M, Kirchhof B, *et al.* (1998) Corneal injury after carbon dioxide laser skin resurfacing. *Am J Ophthal* **125**: 392–394.
9. Blanco G, Soparkar CN, Jordan DR, *et al.* (1999) The ocular complications of periocular laser surgery. *Curr Opin Ophthalmol* **10**: 264–269.
10. Bailey L, Donzis PB, Kastl PR. (1988) Stromal corneal scar following YAG capsulotomy. *Ann Ophthalmol* **20**: 188–190.
11. Alhalel A, Glovinsky Y, Treister G, *et al.* (1993) Long-term follow up of accidental parafoveal laser burns. *Retina* **13**: 152–154.
12. Schmeisser ET. (1993) Acute laser lesion effects on acuity sweep VEPs. *Invest Ophthalmol Vis Sci* **33**: 3546–3554.
13. Park DH, Kim IT. (2009) A case of accidental macular injury by Nd:YAG laser and subsequent 6 year follow-up. *Korean J Ophthalmol* **23**: 207–209.
14. Chuang LH, Lai CC, Yang KJ, *et al.* (2001) A traumatic macular hole secondary to a high-energy Nd:YAG laser. *Ophthalmic Surg Lasers* **32**: 73.
15. Jordan DR. (1986) The potential damaging effects of light on the eye (Part 1). *Can J Ophthalmol* **21**: 216–224.
16. Situm M, Buljan M, Bulat V, *et al.* (2008) The role of UV radiation in the development of basal cell carcinoma. *Coll Antropol* **32**(Suppl. 2): 167–170.
17. Sauter ER, Klein-Szanto AJ, Atillasoy E, *et al.* (1998) Ultraviolet B-induced squamous epithelial and melanocytic cell changes in a xenograft model of cancer development in human skin. *Mol Carcinog* **23**: 168–174.

18. Bigony L. (2007) Risks associated with exposure to surgical smoke plume: a review of the literature. *AORN J* **86**: 1013–1020.
19. Andersen K. (2004) Safe use of lasers in the operating room — what perioperative nurse should know. *AORN J* **79**: 171–188.
20. Yardley IE, Donaldson LJ. (2010) Surgical fires, a clear and present danger. *Surgeon* **8**: 87–92.
21. Prasad R, Quezado Z, St Andre A, *et al.* (2006) Fires in the operating room and intensive care unit: awareness is the key to prevention. *Anesth Analg* **102**: 172–174.
22. Spigelman AD, Swan JR. (2005) Skin antiseptics and the risk of operating theatre fires. *ANZ J Surg* **75**: 556–558.
23. Rinder CS. (2008) Fire safety in the operating room. *Curr Opin Anaesthesiol* **21**: 790–795.
24. Dhepe N. (2009) Recommendations: Minimum standard guidelines of care on requirements for setting up a laser room. *Indian J Dermatol Venereol Leprol* **75**(Suppl. 2): S101–S110.
25. Garden JM, O'Banion MK, Shelnitz LS, *et al.* (1988) Papillomavirus in the vapor of carbon dioxide laser-treated verrucae. *JAMA* **259**: 1199–1202.
26. Sawchuk WS, Weber PJ, Lowy DR, *et al.* (1989) Infectious papillomavirus in the vapor of warts treated with carbon dioxide laser or electrocoagulation: detection and protection. *J Am Acad Dermatol* **21**: 41–49.
27. Garden JM, O'Banion MK, Bakus AD, *et al.* (2002) Viral disease transmitted by laser-generated plume (aerosol). *Arch Dermatol* **138**: 1303–1307.
28. Hallmo P, Naess O. (1991) Laryngeal papillomatosis with human papillomavirus DNA contracted by a laser surgeon. *Eur Arch Otorhinolaryngol* **248**: 425–427.
29. Calero L, Brusis T. (2003) Laryngeal papillomatosis — first recognition in Germany as an occupational disease in an operating room nurse. *Laryngorhinootologie* **82**: 790–793.
30. Plappert UG, Stocker B, Helbig R, *et al.* (1999) Laser pyrolysis products-genotoxic, clastogenic and mutagenic effects of the particulate aerosol fractions. *Mutat Res* **441**: 29–41.
31. Jordan DR. (1986) The potential damaging effects of light on the eye (Part II). *Can J Ophthalmol* **21**: 266–268.
32. Marc REM, Jones BW, Watt CB, *et al.* (2008) Extreme retinal remodeling triggered by light damage: implications for age related macular degeneration. *Mol Vis* **14**: 782–806.

Chapter 3

Carbon Dioxide Laser Surgery in the Asian Skin

Colin Kwok*

Introduction

The carbon dioxide (CO_2) laser was invented by Kumar Patel in 1964 when his research in the pure rare gases led him to discover the laser action of carbon dioxide.[1]

Carbon dioxide lasers come in different configurations. Used conventionally, the laser can be used to cut or coagulate tissue. A scanner may be attached, allowing resurfacing of the skin to be done. This chapter will concentrate on the conventional uses of the CO_2 laser.

Knowing the characteristics of the laser and its tissue interaction is important in adapting the CO_2 laser to treat various skin diseases.

Laser-Tissue Interactions

The CO_2 laser emits light at a wavelength of 10,600 nm in the infrared spectrum. It is absorbed strongly by water, which is found in abundance in the skin. The laser is suitable for treating a wide variety of epidermal and dermal lesions with greater precision than electrosurgery or cryotherapy, but is comparatively more costly.

The theory of selective photothermolysis states that selective heating of the target chromophore can be achieved when using laser pulses shorter than the thermal relaxation time (TRT) of the chromophore.[2] The TRT is the time required for the chromophore to lose 50% of its heat to the surrounding tissue. The TRT for 20–30 micrometers (μm) of skin tissue is approximately 1 millisecond (ms).[3,4]

One pass of the CO_2 laser will vaporize about 20–30 μm of skin in both continuous and pulse mode.[4,5] Beyond this zone of vaporization is a zone of necrosis due to heat conduction from the laser beam.

This zone of necrosis reaches 1 mm in the continuous wave mode (CW). In pulse mode, the zone is narrower, varying from 40–120 μm.[4,5]

The energy fluence (density) necessary to vaporize tissue is approximately 5 J/cm^2 (ablation threshold). By increasing the fluence, one can increase the speed of cutting through the skin tissue.

Advantages of the CO_2 Laser

In pigmented skin, use of other modalities such as cryotherapy may lead to unsightly hypopigmentation due to the melanotoxic effect of extreme cold. This is where the CO_2 laser may offer an advantage.

The thermal heat conduction from the CO_2 laser seals small blood vessels up to 0.5 mm in diameter

*Senior Consultant, Department of Dermatology, Changi General Hospital, Singapore.

and contributes to a bloodless field. The sealing of lymphatics and nerves may contribute to a reduction in tissue swelling and pain.

More recently, the superpulse CO_2 has been shown to enhance wound healing by its effect on dermal cytokines, particularly by stimulating basic fibroblast growth factor (bFGF) and inhibiting transforming growth factor $\beta 1$ (TGF-$\beta 1$) production, and this may be advantageous in the treatment of keloids.[6]

Clinical Applications

Waveform

1. *Continuous wave*

In this mode, the laser acts as a **vaporization device**.

Water in the target tissue absorbs the laser energy, heats up, boils, and vaporizes, taking the surrounding tissue with it.

Approximately 90% of CO_2 laser energy is absorbed in the initial 20–30 μm of the skin. The continuous wave lasers leave behind a thick zone of thermal damage measuring 0.2–1 mm (average 0.5 mm) in thickness.

The continuous wave mode is commonly used to ablate skin lesions such as epidermal nevi and viral warts.

2. *Pulse wave*

The peak power per pulse is 2–10 times that of the continuous wave CO_2 laser but the average power over time is similar.

In this mode, the laser acts as an excision or **cutting device**. The zone of necrosis is thinner compared to the continuous wave mode.

Different laser companies use different terms for the pulse wave.

The Ultrapulse™ (Coherent Medical) produces up to 500 mJ of energy in each pulse measuring 600 microseconds (μs) to 1 ms.[5]

The Tru-Pulse™ (Palomar Medical) delivers 500 mJ at a pulse duration of 60 μs.[5]

The essential principle is by having a pulse duration shorter than the thermal relaxation time of skin (1 ms), minimal damage to the surrounding tissue occurs. This effect is utilized in the excision of skin tissue and in skin resurfacing.

In conclusion, delivering a 1 ms CO_2 laser pulse with an energy fluence of approximately 5 J/cm^2 leads to tissue vaporization to a depth of 20–30 μm and a peripheral zone of thermal injury measuring 40–120 μm.

The pulse mode may be selected to treat small skin lesions such as syringomas or small melanocytic nevi. Here the aim is to limit destruction to the intended lesions with minimal collateral damage.

Spot Size

The CO_2 laser comes with various handpieces of different spot sizes.

For dermatological applications, fixed focus handpieces are ideal, and most have spot sizes less than 1.0 mm in diameter, e.g. 0.15 mm, 0.1 mm, and 0.3 mm. The smaller the spot size, the smaller the area of damage.

The author uses a 0.3 mm spot diameter handpiece which suffices for most conventional CO_2 laser surgery. For smaller lesions, e.g. syringomas, a smaller 0.15 mm spot handpiece may be used.

Defocusing the laser beam by adjusting the distance of the handpiece from the skin allows the operator to vary the spot size. Intra-operatively, if one encounters a bleeding blood vessel, the laser can secure hemostasis by pulling back the handpiece about 1 cm away from the lesion in the defocused mode, thereby converting it to a heating device.

Indications

The CO_2 laser can be used to treat a wide array of dermatological conditions.[7–12]

Epidermal Lesions

Epidermal nevus
Seborrheic keratosis
Viral warts — verruca vulgaris, plane warts

Dermal Lesions

Angiofibroma
Keloid
Rhinophyma
Melanocytic nevus — junctional, compound
Sebaceous hyperplasia
Syringoma
Xanthelesma

Patient Selection

As with all surgical procedures, it is important to select patients with realistic expectations. Avoid patients with psychological instability or unrealistic expectations.

If there are active bacterial, viral, or fungal skin infections, treat the infections first with the appropriate antimicrobial agents.

For facial procedures, especially around the perioral areas, if the patient has a history of herpes labialis infection, start suppressive therapy with oral antiviral medications, e.g. acyclovir 400 mg bd or famiciclovir 250 mg bd or valacyclovir 500 mg once a day two days before the procedure and continue until complete re-epithelialization has taken place.

For patients with a tendency to keloid or hypertrophic scar formation, avoid resurfacing deeper than the papillary dermis.

Patients should have stopped oral isotretinoin for at least six months prior to CO_2 laser surgery.

Delay surgery for at least three months if patient has prior reticular dermis-level resurfacing procedure. Such procedures damage the skin vasculature and time has to be given to allow the vasculature to reform.

In areas poor in adnexal structures, e.g. from previous deep resurfacing procedures or radiation therapy, wound healing may be delayed.

Consider how the scar will appear after healing. For patients with significant lower eyelid laxity, avoid aggressive CO_2 laser resurfacing on the lid to avoid post-resurfacing scleral show and ectropion.

Laser Safety

The following are essential to the safe use of the CO_2 laser:

1. Controlled access to the laser room.
2. Appropriate eye protection for patients, operator, and assistants.
3. Avoidance of inflammable materials, including alcohol-based skin preparations.
4. Non-reflective surgical equipment, e.g. forceps, eye shields.
5. Use of saline-soaked drapes to protect surrounding skin.
6. Use of smoke evacuator. Human papillomavirus DNA and HIV proviral DNA have been isolated in CO_2 generated fumes.[13]

Anesthesia

The majority of CO_2 laser procedures require either topical anesthesia, e.g. EMLA®, or local anesthesia, e.g. 2% lidocaine with or without epinephrine.[7]

In extensive lesions or when the patient is unable to cooperate, general anesthesia may be more suitable.

Side Effects and Complications[5,7]

1. Post-inflammatory Hyperpigmentation

This tends to occur in the darker skin phototypes like the Asian skin. Treating a test spot on a less conspicuous area on the body may help determine if this is likely to occur.

Measures that can be taken to minimize this effect include pre- and post-treatment with broad-spectrum sunscreen, hydroquinone, tretinoin, and avoidance of sun exposure.

Post-inflammatory hyperpigmentation tends to subside over a course of 4–6 months.

2. Post-inflammatory Hypopigmentation

This may be permanent, but fortunately occurs less frequently than hyperpigmentation.

3. Infection

In areas that are relatively clean, e.g. facial lesions, this is usually not a problem. Patients are given topical antibiotics, e.g. tetracycline or mupirocin, to apply to the raw skin until full re-epithelialization.

4. Herpes Simplex Re-activation

If there is a history of recurrent herpes labialis, antiviral prophylaxis is advisable for facial procedures.

5. Scarring

Procedures that ablate lesions below the dermo-epidermal junction, e.g. sebaceous hyperplasia, syringoma etc., will inevitably produce scarring. Patients should be counseled accordingly. For epidermal lesions, deliberate undertreatment may help limit the degree of postoperative scarring. This may translate into additional sessions of laser treatment, but the final appearance will be better. Remember there is a zone of necrosis beyond the zone of vaporization.

6. Postoperative Pain

Most postoperative pain can be managed with the usual oral analgesics, e.g. paracetamol, non-steroidal anti-inflammatory drugs (NSAIDS).

Conclusion

Half a century after its invention, the CO_2 laser remains a useful tool in the armamentarium of the dermatologist.

References

1. Patel CKN. (1964) Continuous-wave laser action on vibraional-rotational transitions of CO_2. *Phys Rev* **136**: A1187–A1193.
2. Anderson RR, Parrish JA. (1988) Selective photothermolysis: precise microsurgery by selective absorption of pulsed radiation. *Science* **220**: 524–527.
3. McKenzie AL. (1983) How far does thermal damage extend beneath the surface of CO_2 laser incisions. *Phys Med Bio* **28**: 905–912.
4. Lou WW, Geronemus RG. (2002) Dermatologic laser surgery. *Sem Cutan Med Surg* **21**: 107–128.
5. Alexiades-Armenakas MR, Dover JS, Arndt KA. (2008) The spectrum of laser skin resurfacing: nonablative, fractional, and ablative laser resurfacing. *J Am Acad Dermatol* **58**: 719–739.
6. Novak KC, McCormack M, Koch RJ. (2000) The effect of superpulsed carbon dioxide laser energy on keloid and normal dermal fibroblast secretion of growth factors: a serum-free study. *Plast Reconstr Surg* **105**: 2039–2048.

7. Tanzi EL, Lupton JR, Alster TS. (2003) Lasers in dermatology: four decades of progress. *J Am Acad Dermatol* **49**: 1–31.
8. Markus RF. (2000) Lasers: more than a cosmetic tool. *J Dermatol Treat* **11**: 117–124.
9. Sinclair RJ, Sinclair PJ. (1992) Carbon dioxide laser in the treatment of cutaneous disorders. *Australas J Dermatol* **32**: 165–171.
10. Sood S, Hruza GJ. (2000) Treatment of verruca vulgaris and condyloma acuminatum with lasers. *Dermatol Ther* **13**: 90–101.
11. Logan RA, Zachary CB. (1989) Outcome of carbon dioxide laser therapy for persistent cutaneous viral warts. *Br J Dermatol* **121**: 99–105.
12. Morosolli ARC, Cardoso GDOM, LM Santos, *et al.* (2008) Surgical treatment of earlobe keloid with CO_2 laser radiation: case report and clinical standpoints. *J Cosmet Laser Ther* **10**: 226–230.
13. Goyal S, Dover JS, Arndt KA. (1995) Lasers. *J Am Acad Dermatol* **32**: 262–272.

Carbon Dioxide Laser in Selected Skin Disorders

Epidermal Nevus

Case 1: A Malay teenager has an epidermal nevus at the left corner of his mouth since birth. It has gradually grown in size over the years.

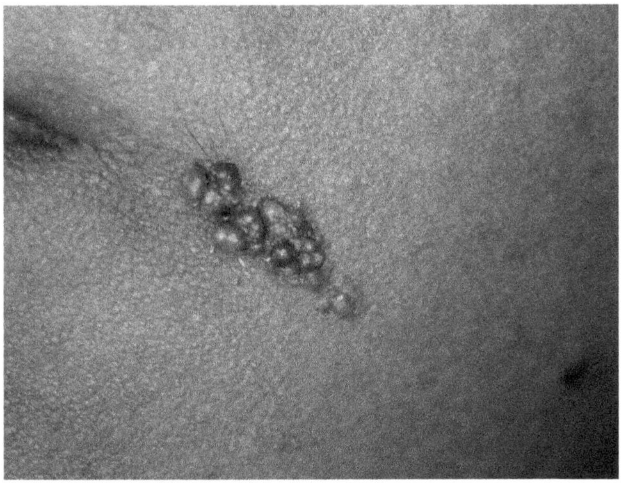

Figure 3.1.

Case 1. Epidermal nevus.

Topical EMLA® was used as anesthesia. Local anesthesia may be given in addition but was not needed in this case.

CO_2 laser parameters: 0.3 mm spot size, continuous wave, fluence 5 J/cm^2. The laser beam was painted to and fro on the nevus to ablate it to the level of the surrounding skin using continuous mode. In continuous mode, the laser keeps firing as long as the foot pedal is depressed and is useful for rapid ablation of cutaneous lesions.

Towards the end of the procedure, the mode was changed to repeat mode, where the frequency of firing is less rapid compared to continuous mode, thus allowing greater precision.

There was a deliberate attempt to undertreat so as to reduce scar formation.

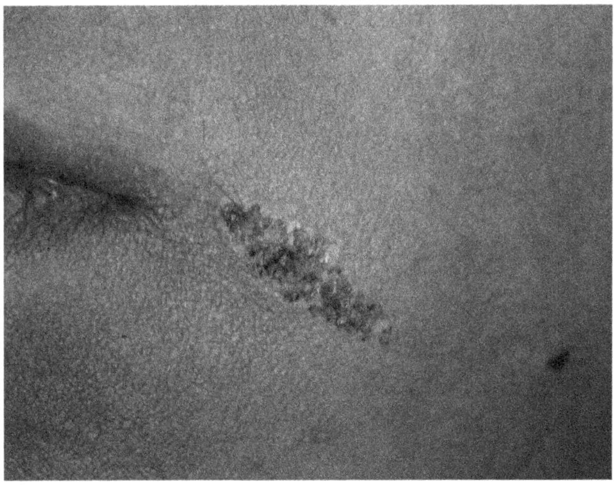

Figure 3.2.

Immediate post laser.

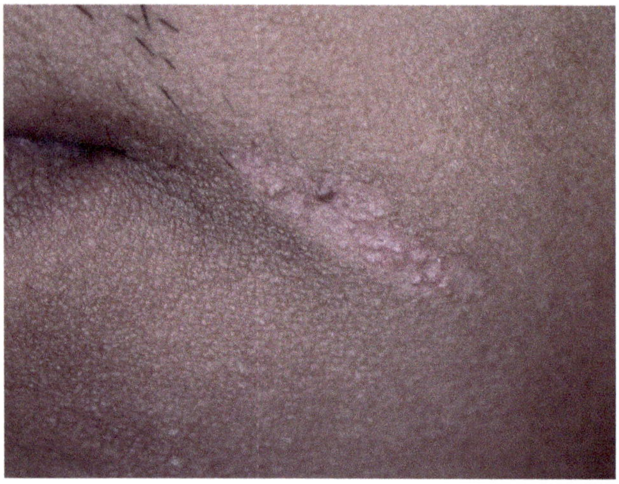

Figure 3.3.

Three months post laser.

The laser wound healed well, with marked cosmetic improvement. There was slight hypopigmentation and minimal scarring.

Keloids

Keloids may occur after surgical removal, especially if they occur in areas of the body subjected to repeated stretching/tension of the skin, e.g. on the chest.

Case 2: This young girl had her ear pierced but developed a keloid on her left earlobe.

Local anesthesia (2% lidocaine with epinephrine) was given.

The CO_2 laser was used with superpulse wave using a fluence of 7 J/cm^2 to excise the base of keloid, taking care to stay within the borders of the keloid.

Subsequently, the laser was switched to continuous wave while maintaining the same fluence, and the surface of the cut keloid was painted to level it.

The wound healed well. An intralesional steroid injection (triamcinolone acetonide, 40 mg/ml) was given into the base to prevent keloid formation, starting one month post laser treatment. Alternatively, intralesional steroids may be injected at the time of laser ablation. The injection may be repeated monthly and the interval gradually lengthened depending on the response.

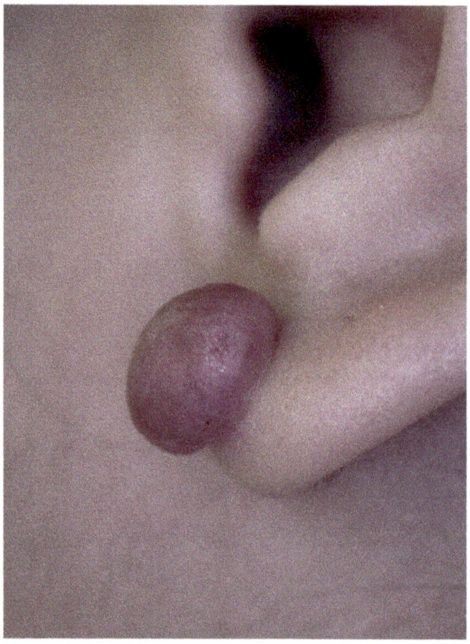

Figure 3.4.

Case 2. Keloid left earlobe.

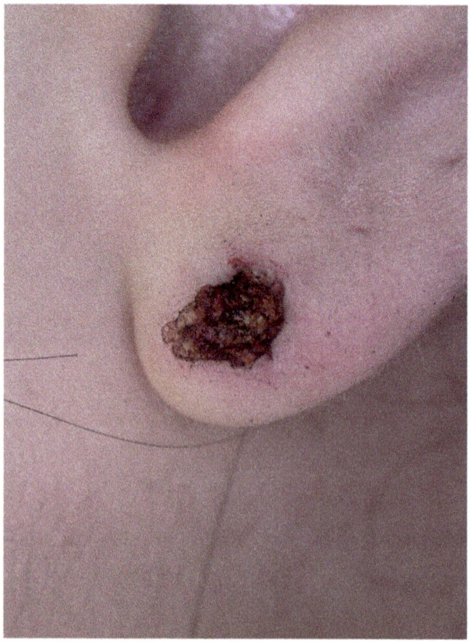

Figure 3.5.

Immediate post-operation.

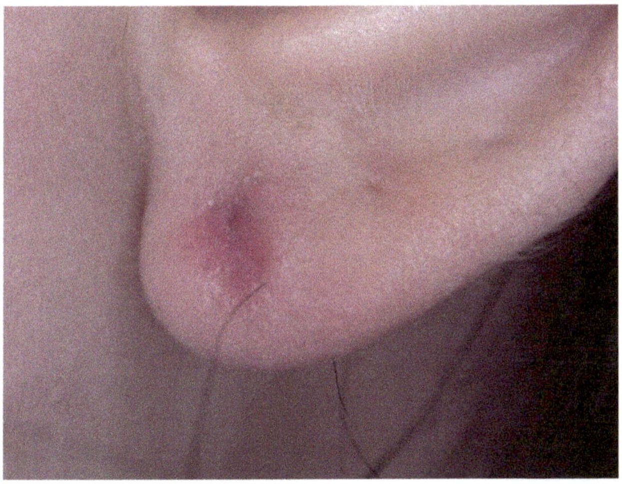

Figure 3.6.

One month post-operation.

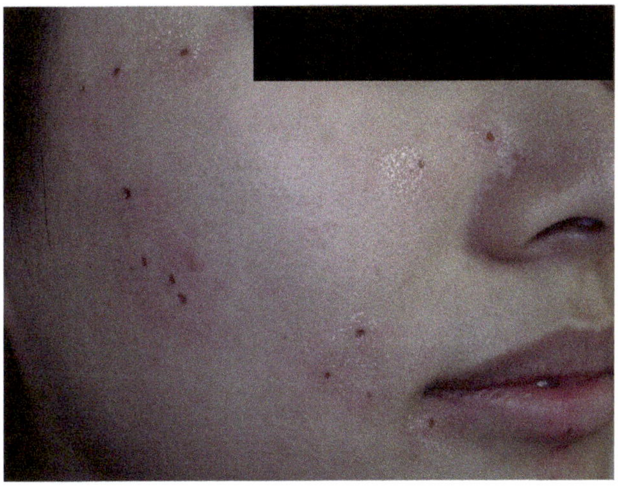

Figure 3.8.

Immediate post-operation.

Melanocytic Nevi

Case 3: This Chinese girl had been teased because of the unsightly appearance of her facial moles.

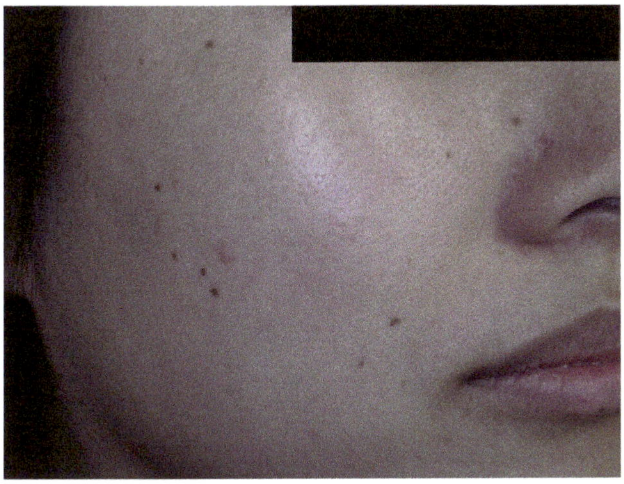

Figure 3.7.

Case 3. Facial junctional melanocytic nevi.

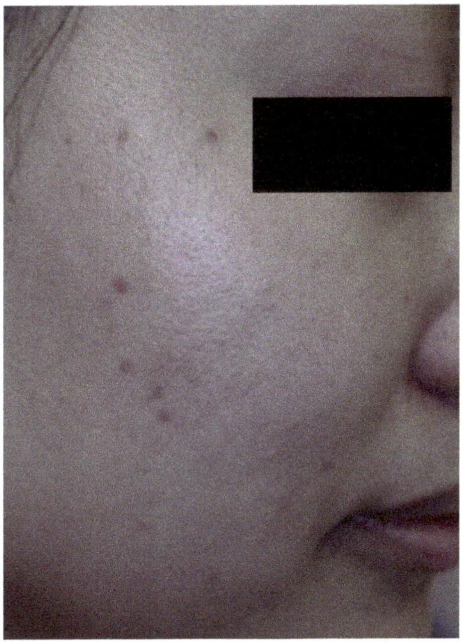

Figure 3.9.

One month post-operation.

Local anesthesia (2% lidocaine with epinephrine) was given to each site of operation.

CO_2 laser parameters: 0.3 mm spot size, superpulse wave, fluence 5 J/cm^2. Superpulse was used to limit surrounding tissue necrosis and ultimately the size of subsequent scarring.

The wounds had partially re-epithelialized, with mild erythema and slight depression.

Recalcitrant Plantar Wart

Case 4: This elderly Indian man had a persistent right plantar wart for many years, which had failed multiple sessions of cryotherapy.

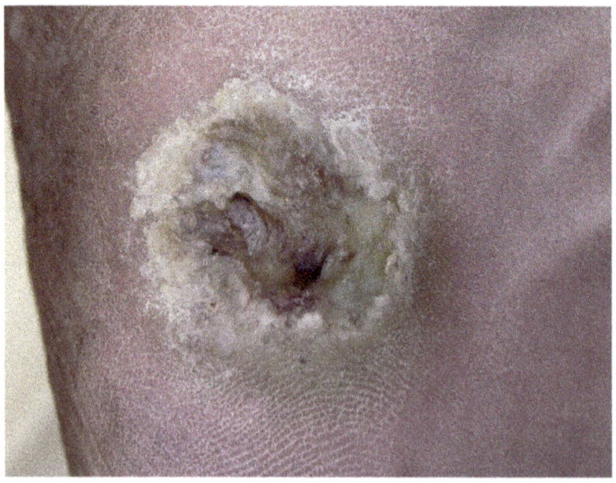

Figure 3.10.

Case 4. Plantar wart.

An ice pack was applied to the skin at the sites of injection for several seconds before injection of local anesthesia (2% lidocaine with epinephrine). This helped reduce the pain of the injection.

The hyperkeratotic area was first pared down with a scalpel.

The CO_2 laser was set at continuous wave at a fluence of 10 J/cm^2.

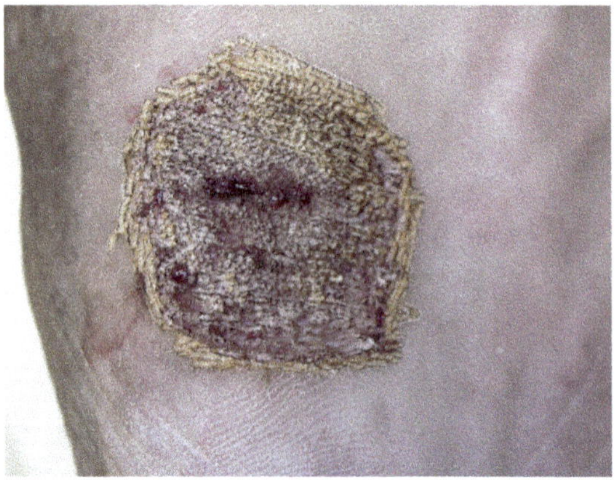

Figure 3.11.

Immediate post-operation.

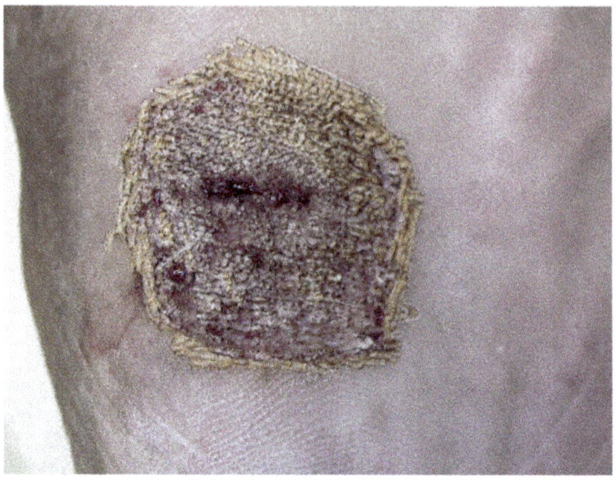

Figure 3.12.

One month after laser.

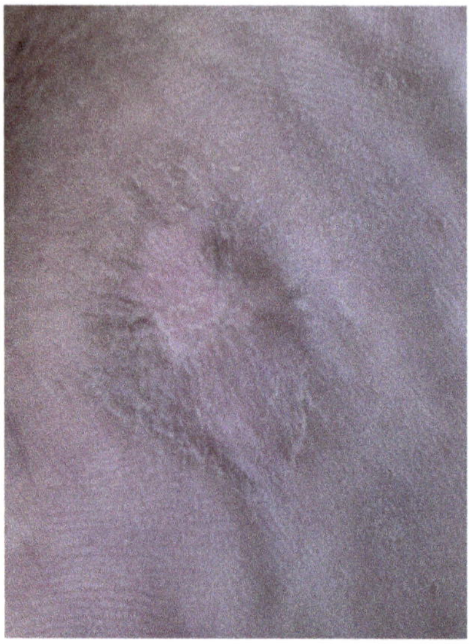

Figure 3.13.

Three months post laser.

The wart was lasered down to the papillary dermis, together with a rim of about 5 mm of normal appearing skin.

The wound eventually healed with a depressed scar and no residual wart.

Syringomata

Case 5: A middle-aged Chinese woman wanted to remove her unsightly syringomas.

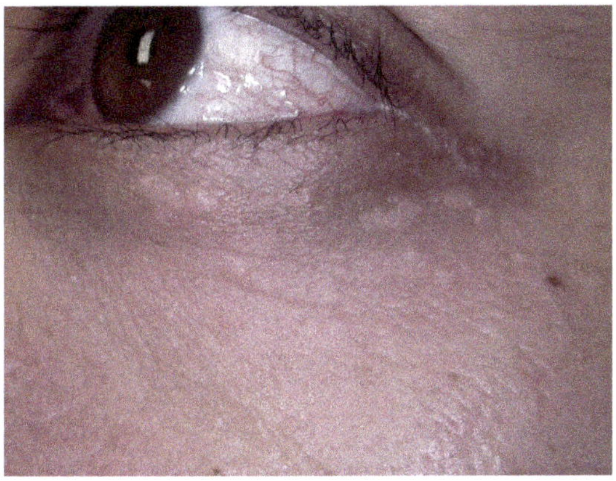

Figure 3.14.

Case 5. Syringomas left periorbital area.

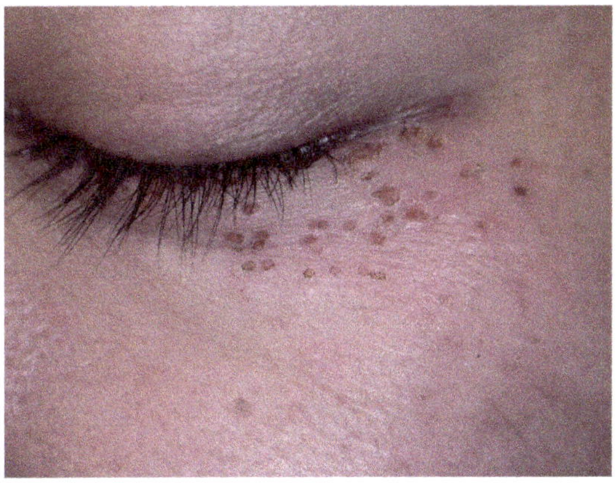

Figure 3.15.

Immediate post-operation.

EMLA® was applied to the area. Additional 2% lidocaine with epinephrine may be given but this patient did not require it.

A handpiece with a smaller spot size 0.15 mm was used.

Here, precision was important to limit the lasering to the intended area and to avoid collateral damage. Superpulse wave was selected at a fluence of 5 J/cm^2.

Eye protection was essential. The metal eye goggle had to be carefully shifted as the procedure progressed, keeping the eye covered throughout.

An alternative eye protection would be to use an intra-ocular eye shield.

The operating hand was further stabilized by resting on the non-operating hand.

The wounds healed with mild scarring and hypopigmentation. Her facial appearance had improved compared to before the operation.

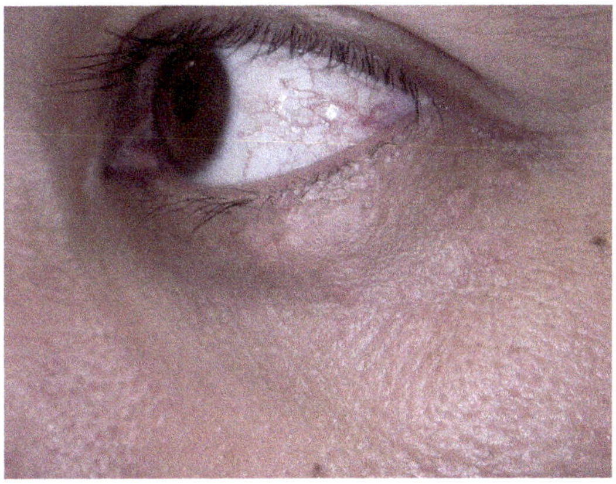

Figure 3.16.

One month post-operation.

Chapter 4

Vascular Lasers in the Asian Skin

Yuin-Chew Chan*

Introduction

Lasers can be used to treat congenital and acquired vascular lesions (Table 4.1), based on the principle of selective photothermolysis.[1,2]

Vascular Lasers and Light Sources

Several lasers and light sources are useful in the treatment of vascular lesions (Table 4.2). These include:

— pulsed potassium-titanyl-phosphate (KTP) laser
— pulsed dye laser
— alexandrite laser
— diode laser
— long-pulsed Nd:YAG laser
— intense pulsed light (IPL)

To select appropriate laser parameters, it is important to have an idea of the size and depth of the target vessels:

$<$ 1 mm depth: green or yellow light
$<$ 2 mm depth: red light
$<$ 4 mm depth: near-infrared light

Wavelength

Oxyhemoglobin is the target chromophore. By specifically targeting and heating oxyhemoglobin, vascular endothelial cells are damaged. The three major peaks in oxyhemoglobin absorption occur within the visible spectrum, at 418 nm, 542 nm, and 577 nm. Since melanin competes with oxyhemoglobin at these wavelengths, it is important to select a wavelength that is significantly better absorbed by oxyhemoglobin than by melanin. Interference by epidermal melanin may result in dyspigmentation (hypo- and hyperpigmentation) that lasts for weeks to months.

The wavelength used has to achieve sufficient penetration into the skin to reach the target vessel. Longer wavelengths penetrate deeper, but require higher fluences for efficacy. Skin cooling is important to avoid damage to the epidermis.

Lasers with wavelengths from 532–1064 nm are used to treat vascular lesions. The infrared lasers, i.e. alexandrite (755 nm), diode (800, 940 nm), and Nd:YAG (1064 nm), can penetrate deeper, up to 5 mm below the dermal-epidermal junction. They are useful for the treatment of telangiectasia, venulectasia, and reticular veins, and for reducing the volume of bulky vascular lesions like hemangiomas and venous malformations.

In the author's experience, IPL (550–1400 nm) with a large spot size and absorption by oxy- and deoxyhemoglobin is useful for the treatment of vessel matting, but caution should be exercised in dark or suntanned skin.

Pulse Duration (Pulse Width)

A laser pulse with a duration shorter than the thermal relaxation time of the target and with adequate fluence will destroy the target, with minimal heat

*Consultant Dermatologist, Dermatology Associates, Gleneagles Medical Centre, Singapore.

Table 4.1.

Lesions Amenable to Vascular Laser Treatment

Congenital Vascular Lesions
Hemangioma
Vascular malformations
— capillary (port wine stain)
— venous
Acquired Vascular Lesions
Telangiectasia
Angioma
Pyogenic granuloma
Venous lake
Leg veins
Angiofibroma
Angiokeratoma
Poikiloderma of Civatte
Miscellaneous Lesions
Hypertrophic scar/keloid
Viral wart

damage to the surrounding tissue. The optimal pulse duration depends on the diameter of the target vessel.

$$\text{Thermal relaxation} = (\text{vessel diameter})^2/4k$$

where k is thermal diffusivity.

Optimum pulse duration for treatment of vascular lesions lies in the millisecond (ms) range, usually about 1–100 ms.

At longer pulse durations, the heat produced by the laser is spread over a longer duration of time and heats the vessel more gently. This reduces vessel rupture and produces less purpura than shorter pulse durations.

Hence, lasers with longer pulse durations are used to treat larger and deeper vessels like leg veins and large vascular anomalies. Lasers with shorter pulse durations are suitable for port wine stains and small, superficial telangiectasias on the face.

Fluence

This is selected based on the clinical endpoint specific for each laser and for the particular disease entity. Clinical endpoints include purpura, vessel blanching or clearance, and erythema.

Epidermal Cooling

Skin cooling is important for several reasons:

- — to cool the epidermis and protect it from damage, hence allowing the use of higher fluences, resulting in more effective treatment.
- — to reduce the pain associated with the laser treatment.

Cooling strategies include cryogen spray and contact cooling (chilled tips, cooled glass chambers, sapphire windows).

Vascular Laser Treatment in Infants and Children

Anesthesia is an important consideration when laser therapy is used in infants and children.

Table 4.2.

Lasers and Light Sources for the Treatment of Vascular Lesions

Laser	Wavelength (nm)	Pulse Duration (ms)	Treatment Endpoint
Pulsed KTP	532	1–200	Erythema, edema
Pulsed dye laser	585–595	0.45–10	Purpura
Alexandrite	755	5–20	Vessel blanching, purpura
Diode	800, 940	5–250	Vessel blanching
Long pulsed Nd:YAG	1064	20–50	Vessel blanching
Intense pulsed light (IPL)	550–1400	8–50	Purpura, erythema, or edema

Topical Anesthesia

EMLA® cream is a eutectic mixture of 2.5% lidocaine and 2.5% prilocaine. It is applied under occlusion for one hour before the laser procedure. The maximum recommended doses for EMLA® cream on intact healthy skin in children are shown in Table 4.3. As EMLA® cream commonly causes blanching of vascular lesions, it is helpful to outline the lesions with a skin marker before application. Peri-orbital application should be avoided as corneal ulceration and irritation are possible adverse effects if the cream is accidentally rubbed into the eyes. Methemo-globinemia due to the prilocaine component has been reported, mainly in neonates less than three months of age, as their methemoglobin reductase pathway is immature.[3]

Liposomal lignocaine (LMX®) is a topical anesthetic that is encapsulated in a phospholipid-based carrier. Liposomal vehicles facilitate diffusion of lignocaine through the dermis. In comparative clinical trials, LMX® (applied for 30 min) and EMLA® (applied for 60 min) were equally effective in reducing pain in children.[4,5] The faster onset of anesthesia with LMX® is an advantage in pediatric practice. There have been no reports of serious adverse effects with the use of LMX®. However, LMX® should not be applied for longer than two hours to avoid excessive systemic levels of lignocaine. In children lighter than 20 kg, liposomal lignocaine should not be applied to a surface area greater than 100 cm^2.[6]

The absence of prilocaine eliminates the risk of methemoglobinemia.

Table 4.3.

Recommended EMLA® Dosing on Intact and Healthy Skin in Children[10]

Age/Body Weight	Maximum Dose (g)	Maximum Application Area (cm²)	Maximum Application Time (h)
0–3 mth old or <5 kg	1	10	1
2–12 mth old and >5 kg	2	20	4
1–6 yr old and >10 kg	10	100	4
7–12 yr old and >20 kg	20	200	4

General Anesthesia

An increased risk of complications is associated with the use of general anesthesia in the first year of life, with an even greater risk in the first month of life.[7–9] Hence, it would be prudent to avoid general anesthesia in young infants as far as possible.

Eye Protection

The standard eye goggles are too large and poorly fitting for infants and young children. The use of 2 to 3 layers of moist white gauze to cover the eyes is a good alternative. Pediatric metal corneal shields should be used if the peri-orbital skin is treated.

Port Wine Stains

This is a benign congenital capillary malformation that occurs sporadically with an incidence rate of about 0.3–0.5%.[11] Histologically, it is composed of ectatic capillaries in the superficial dermis. At birth, it is macular and pink. As the child grows older, it becomes darker (red or purple) and may develop vascular nodularity or soft tissue hypertrophy if left untreated. The lesion does not involute spontaneously.

Laser treatment is often started in early childhood to prevent these complications. Early treatment also results in more rapid clearing. The pulsed dye laser, which emits yellow light, is the gold standard for the treatment of port wine stains. Typical parameters are spot size 7–10 mm, pulse duration 0.45–1.5 ms, and fluence 6–12 J/cm^2. Treatment is repeated at 1–2-monthly intervals. Port wine stains around the eyes, on the forehead, temple, lateral cheeks, chin, and neck respond better compared to those on the central cheeks, nose, and

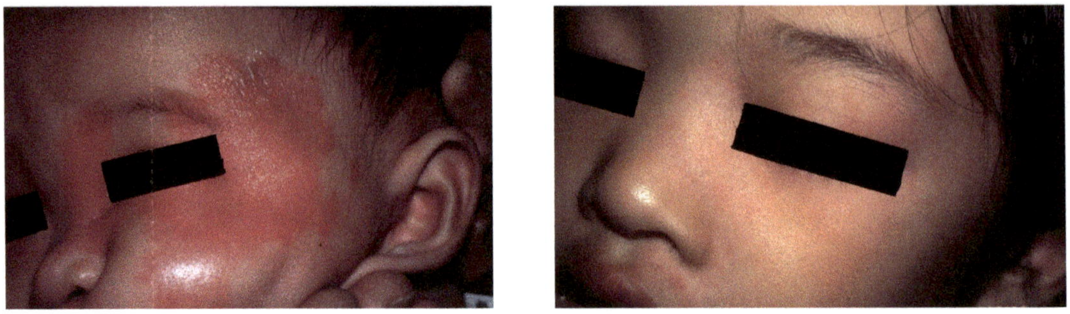

(a) (b)

Figure 4.1.

Case 1. Port wine stain. (a) Before treatment. (b) After 8 treatments at 2–4 month intervals with the 595 nm pulsed dye laser showing significant lightening: 7 mm spot, 10–12.5 J/cm^2, 1.5 ms pulse duration, 40 ms cryogen spray with a 20 ms delay. (Courtesy of Tay YK, FRCP, Singapore.)

upper lip.[12] Port wine stains on the proximal limb respond faster than those on the distal limb.[13]

Most children achieve about 55% lightening after the first five treatment sessions and 18% improvement with the next five sessions.[14] A series of 6–12 treatment sessions are required to achieve significant lightening (Fig. 4.1).

More treatment sessions are usually required in adults. Potential side effects of the pulsed dye laser treatment include hyperpigmentation, hypopigmentation, and scarring.

In a retrospective study, 94 Asian patients (skin types III and IV), mean age 26.4 years (range 1–58 years), experienced good to excellent responses after an average of four treatment sessions using the 585 nm pulsed dye laser.[15]

Vascular nodules or blebs in adults can be ablated with the carbon dioxide laser or electrosurgery first, before proceeding with vascular laser therapy of the port wine stain. Hypertrophic port wine stains in adults may require treatment with the long-pulsed 1064 nm Nd:YAG laser[16] or 755 nm alexandrite laser,[17] as the longer wavelengths allow for deeper penetration. However, caution (adequate skin cooling, starting at more conservative fluences, avoiding overlapping pulses) must be exercised with these lasers to avoid ulceration and scarring.

A prospective trial was performed involving 22 Chinese patients (ages 6–45 years, mean age 21.8 years) with untreated port wine stains. They each received 5–7 sessions of IPL therapy at intervals of 3–4 weeks.[18] Fifty percent of patients had 25–50% clearing and 40% of patients showed more than 50% clinical clearance. The only two patients with less than 25% clearing had nodular port wine stains. The procedures were well tolerated. One patient developed blisters, but none had any long-term complications.[18] Other studies have shown that IPL can be useful in treating port wine stains that were resistant to previous pulsed dye laser therapy.[19]

Case 2

A 30-year-old Chinese female with pulsed-dye-laser-resistant port wine stain on the left cheek was treated with IPL, wavelength 555–950 nm, pulse duration 8 ms, fluence 15–16 J/cm^2, single pulsing, using nonoverlapping pulses, at 2-monthly intervals (Fig. 4.2).

Hemangiomas

This is a benign vascular tumor characterized by endothelial cell hyperproliferation that appears within the first eight weeks of life. It is less common in Asian infants as compared to Caucasian infants.[20] It proliferates during the first 6–9 months of age and

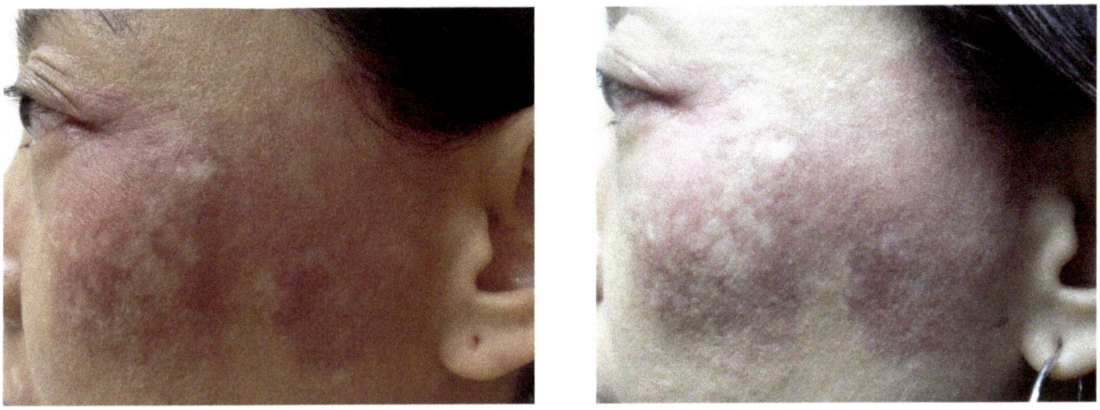

(a) (b)

Figure 4.2.

Case 2. Port wine stain. (a) Before treatment. (b) After 3 treatment sessions, showing signfcant lightening of the port wine stain with the IPL.

subsequently involutes, usually after the first year of life. However, even with complete involution, the skin may not return to normal. Up to 50% of hemangiomas have some residual telangiectasia or fibrofatty change. Hemangiomas may be superficial, subcutaneous, or mixed tumors.

Most hemangiomas do not require treatment and can be observed for spontaneous involution. However, some may be life- or function-threatening or cosmetically disfiguring, and thus require treatment.

Laser treatment can be considered under the following circumstances:

— Ulcerated hemangioma. This is painful, often bleeds and may become secondarily infected. If it is located on the lip or the anogenital region, the pain may lead to problems with feeding, micturition, or defecation.
— Superficial hemangioma that is cosmetically disfiguring.
— Residual telangiectasia that persists after involution of the hemangioma.

The pulsed dye laser is the treatment of choice. Subpurpuric fluences are used to avoid causing ulceration. Hemangiomas assessed to be suitable for treatment should be treated early in an attempt to reduce proliferation. Limited penetration of the pulsed dye laser, up to a depth of about 1.2 mm, makes the treatment of deep hemangiomas ineffective.[21]

Typical parameters for pulsed dye laser treatment of hemangiomas are spot size 7–10 mm, pulse duration 1.5 ms, fluence 5–8 J/cm^2. Potential side effects of pulsed dye laser treatment include scabbing and ulceration (which may result in scarring and hypopigmentation).

A randomized controlled study of 121 infants aged 1–14 weeks with early hemangiomas suggested that pulsed dye laser treatment in uncomplicated hemangiomas is not better than observation.[22] Possible reasons for this and the higher incidence of scarring in the treatment group include the use of high fluences and absence of dynamic cooling.

Case 3

A 2-month-old female infant presented with an infected ulcerated hemangioma on the lower lip. Management included wound care with normal saline wash and mupirocin ointment, control of infection with oral amoxicillin, pain relief with lignocaine gel, and suppression of proliferation with oral prednisolone 1 mg/kg/day. She was also treated with

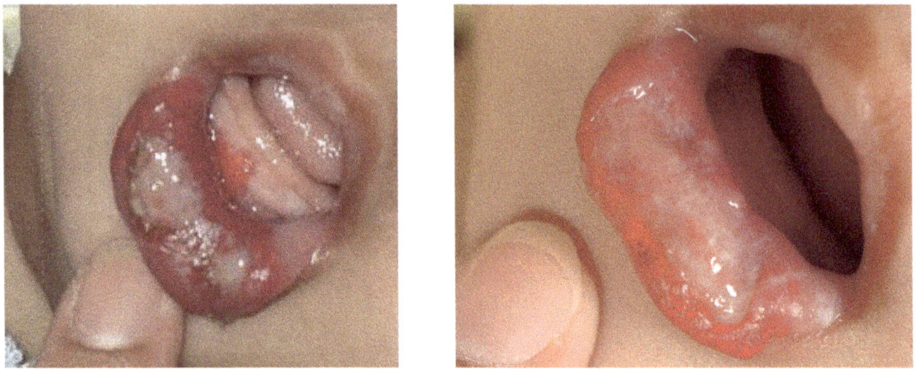

(a) (b)

Figure 4.3.

Case 3. Ulcerated hemangioma. (a) Before treatment. (b) At 3 weeks, after 2 treatment sessions, showing healing of the ulceration.

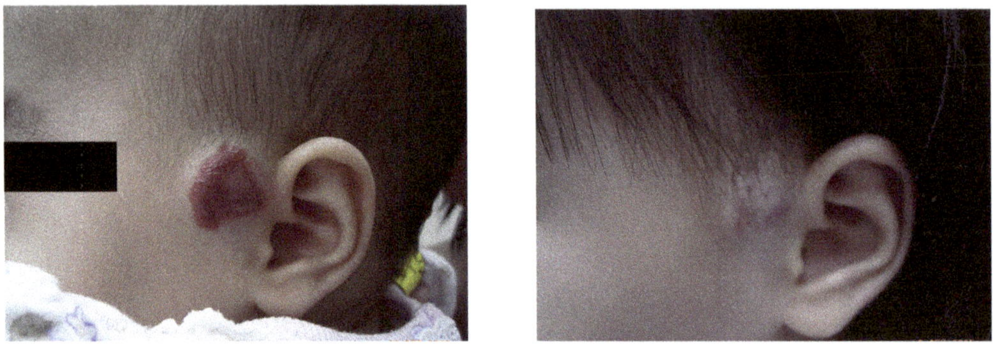

(a) (b)

Figure 4.4.

Case 4. Mixed hemangioma. (a) Before treatment. (b) After 7 treatments at 2–4 week intervals with the 595 nm pulsed dye laser showing significant lightening: 7 mm spot, 10–12 J/cm^2, 1.5 ms pulse duration, 40 ms cryogen spray with a 20 ms delay. (Courtesy of Tay YK, FRCP, Singapore.)

the 595 nm pulsed dye laser, spot size 7 mm, pulse duration 1.5 ms, fluence 8–9 J/cm^2 at 2-weekly intervals. The ulcerated hemangioma healed with atrophic scarring after three weeks (Fig. 4.3).

Telangiectasias

This may be caused by actinic damage, rosacea, connective tissue disease, hepatic dysfunction, or trauma. Histology reveals dilated post-capillary venules with thickened vessel walls and diameters between 0.2 and 0.5 mm in the upper dermis.

The pulsed dye laser is effective for treating telangiectases, with excellent therapeutic outcome. The endpoint is immediate vessel coagulation or clearance, followed by purpura. Longer pulse durations can be used to minimize purpura, but may be slower in clearing telangiectasia. Typical parameters are spot size 7 mm, pulse duration 6–10 ms, fluence 9–12 J/cm^2. Double- or triple-pulse stacking can be used with caution in vessels that refill after the initial pulse.

Case 5

A 25-year-old Indian woman with nasal telangiectases was treated with the 595 nm pulsed dye laser, 7 mm spot size, 6 ms pulse duration, fluence 10 J/cm^2, with double-pulse stacking. This resulted in total clearance of the telangiectases but she developed post-laser hyperpigmentation that lasted several weeks (Fig. 4.5).

Spider Angiomas

These are also known as spider nevi or spider telangiectasias. They contain a central feeder arteriole, diameter about 0.1–0.5 mm, with superficial branches that radiate outwards. Spider angiomas are usually found on the sun-exposed skin, e.g. face, neck, chest, and arms. They respond well to pulsed dye laser therapy, usually requiring 1–2 treatment sessions to clear. Typical parameters are spot size 7 mm, pulse duration 1.5–6 ms, and fluence 9–12 J/cm^2. Double- or triple-pulse stacking can be used with caution.

Cherry Angiomas

These are benign vascular tumors that appear as small red papules, usually on the trunk in adults.

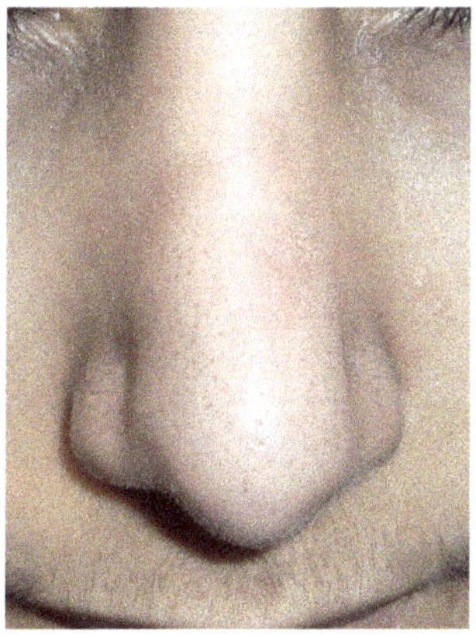

Figure 4.5.

Case 5. Post-laser hyperpigmentation that lasted for several weeks and resolved with sun protection.

Therapeutic options include electrosurgery, cryotherapy, and vascular laser therapy. The pulsed dye laser provides an effective and safe treatment, and usually eradicates the lesion in 1–2 treatment sessions. Typical parameters are similar to those used in the treatment of spider angiomas. As the size of the cherry angioma is smaller than the spot size of the pulsed dye laser, it is useful to isolate the lesion with a white and moist template to protect the surrounding skin.

Pyogenic Granulomas

These benign vascular tumors present as red papules that are prone to bleeding or ulceration. They occur more commonly in childhood. Histologically, the early lesion has numerous capillaries and venules, with plump endothelial cells arrayed radially toward the skin surface in an edematous stroma containing a mixed inflammatory infiltrate, with overlying erosion or ulceration. The mature lesion shows a fibromyxoid stroma separating the lesion into lobules. Shave excision with electrodessication of the base or scalpel excision is often curative. The pulsed dye laser can be considered a fairly effective and safe treatment for small pyogenic granulomas in children who are afraid or unable to cooperate with surgical excision.[23] Typical parameters are spot size 7 mm, pulse duration 1.5–6 ms, and fluence 10–12 J/cm^2. Double- or triple-pulse stacking can be used cautiously.

Leg Veins

Patients with deep venous disease or insufficiency should first be referred to the vascular surgeon for assessment and treatment before embarking on treatment of the superficial spider and small reticular veins.

Therapeutic options for superficial spider and small reticular veins include sclerotherapy and vascular laser therapy. Lasers suitable for treating leg veins include the long-pulsed Nd:YAG (1064 nm)[24,25] diode laser[26] and pulsed dye laser (595 nm).[27]

The long pulse duration (10–100 ms) of the Nd:YAG laser allows selective heating of larger vessels with relative sparing of finer vessels (which tend to cool faster). When compared to the pulsed dye laser, the longer wavelength of the Nd:YAG laser allows deeper penetration. However, there is limited absorption by hemoglobin at 1064 nm, and hence high fluences are required. Small spot sizes (e.g. 2.5 mm) allow such high fluences (100–200 J/cm^2) to be attained, and also limit collateral damage to the surrounding tissue.[25]

Fine spider veins on the legs respond well to the pulsed dye laser. Typical parameters are spot size 7 mm, pulse duration 6–10 ms, and fluence 10–14 J/cm^2. Double- or triple-pulse stacking can be used with caution. However, post-inflammatory hyperpigmentation is common in the Asian skin.

Case 6

A 40-year-old female with fine spider veins on her legs was treated with the 595 nm pulsed dye laser, spot size 7 mm, pulse duration 10 ms, fluence 12 J/cm^2, with double-pulse stacking (Fig. 4.6).

Viral Warts

The pulsed dye laser has been reported to be effective in the treatment of recalcitrant viral warts.[28,29] The mechanism of action is unclear, but may be a result of the intense heating of dermal vessels with collateral damage to viral-infected keratinocytes. Typical parameters are spot size 7 mm, pulse duration 1.5 ms, fluence 12–14 J/cm^2, and double or triple pulsing.

Hypertrophic Scars/Keloids

A few studies have reported significant improvement in erythema and thickness of scars treated with the pulsed dye laser. The mechanism of action may be an effect on collagen following ischemia due to photothermolysis of blood vessels. Typical parameters are spot size 7–10 mm, pulse duration 0.45–6 ms,

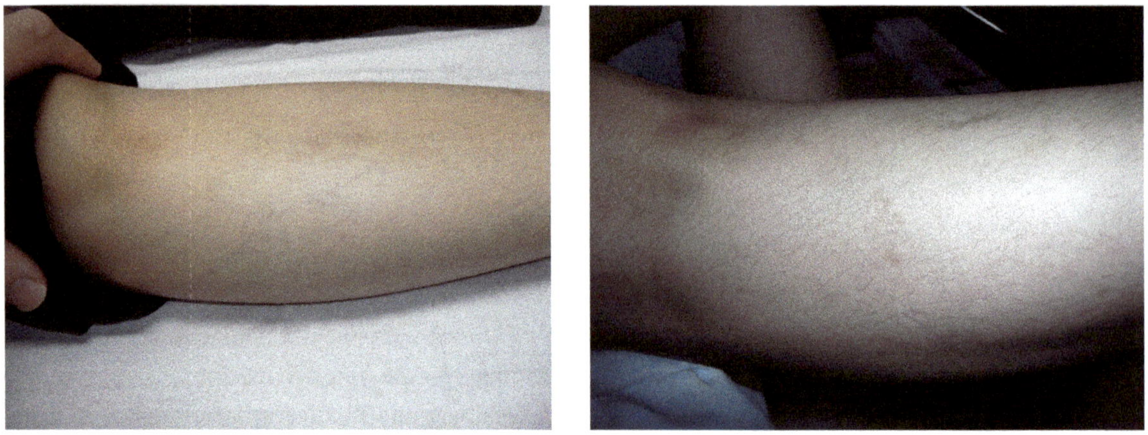

(a) (b)

Figure 4.6.

Case 6. Fine spider leg veins. (a) Before treatment. (b) After 1 treatment session, clearance of the fine spider veins was achieved, but mild post-inflammatory hyperpigmentation remained 1 mth after treatment.

fluence 5–9 J/cm^2, double pulsing, with a shorter pulse duration, e.g. 0.45 ms, being more effective than a longer pulse width, e.g. 40 ms.[30]

Postoperative Care

Cooling the treated skin with a damp cloth that has been soaked in cold water provides immediate postoperative pain relief. Photoprotection and use of sunscreen are important to reduce the risk of post-inflammatory hyperpigmentation. The patient is advised to gently cleanse and moisturize the treated skin, and to expect the purpura to resolve within 1–2 weeks.

Side Effects and Complications

Post-inflammatory hyperpigmentation may occur due to excessive cryogen spray, high laser energies, or excessive exposure to sunlight, especially in skin phototypes V and VI. It may last several weeks to months, but is expected to resolve spontaneously.

Blistering and scabbing may occur if there is inadequate peri-operative skin cooling or high fluences are used. Meticulous skin care with prophylactic topical antibiotics will often suffice. Ulceration and scarring are rare in the hands of the experienced laser surgeon.

Conclusion

Congenital and acquired vascular lesions can be safely and effectively treated with the vascular lasers, even in the pediatric population. Topical anesthesia can be used but may blanch vascular lesions, and may be omitted in adult patients. Patients must be warned of postoperative purpura that may last up to three weeks. Longer pulse durations can be used to reduce or avoid purpura, but may be less effective in clearing vascular lesions. Asian patients may experience postoperative pigmentary changes that may last up to several months. Peri-operative epidermal cooling and postoperative photoprotection help to reduce the risk of adverse effects.

References

1. Anderson RR, Parrish JA. (1981) Microvasculature can be selectively damaged using dye lasers: a basic theory and experimental evidence in human skin. *Lasers Surg Med* **1**: 263–276.
2. Anderson RR, Parrish JA. (1983) Selective photothermolysis: precise microsurgery by selective absorption of pulsed radiation. *Science* **220**: 524–527.
3. Jakobson B, Nilsson A. (1985) Methemoglobinemia in children treated with prilocaine–lidocaine cream and trimethoprim-suphamethoxazole. A case report. *Acta Anaesth Scand* **29**: 453–455.
4. Eichenfield LF, Funk A, Fallon-Friedlander S, *et al.* (2002) A clinical study to evaluate the efficacy of ELA-Max (4% liposomal lidocaine) as compared with eutectic mixture of local anesthetics cream for pain reduction of venipuncture in children. *Pediatrics* **109**: 1093–1099.
5. Kleiber C, Sorenson M, Whiteside K, *et al.* (2002) Topical anesthetics for intravenous insertion in children: a randomized equivalency study. *Pediatrics* **110**: 758–761.
6. Friedman PM, Mafong EA, Friedman ES, *et al.* (2001) Topical anesthetics update: EMLA and beyond. *Dermatol Surg* **27**: 1019–1026.
7. Tiret L, Nivoche Y, Hatton F, *et al.* (1988) Complications related to anaesthesia in infants and children. A prospective survey of 40,240 anaesthetics. *Br J Anaesth* **61**: 263–269.
8. Holzman RS. (1994) Morbidity and mortality in pediatric anesthesia. *Pediatr Clin N Am* **41**: 239–256.
9. Cohen MM, Cameron CB, Duncan PG. (1990) Pediatric anesthesia morbidity and mortality in the perioperative period. *Anesth Analg* **70**: 160–167.
10. Yeo LF, Eichenfield LF, Chan YC. (2007) Skin surgery in children: local anaesthesia and sedation techniques. *Expert Opin Pharmacother* **8**: 317–327.

11. Stratigos AJ, Dover JS, Arndt KA. (2007) Laser therapy. In: Bolognia JL, Jorizzo JL, Rapini RP (eds.), *Dermatology*, pp. 2153–2176. Mosby, London.
12. Renfro L, Geronemus RG. (1993) Anatomical differences of port-wine stains in response to treatment with the pulsed dye laser. *Arch Dermatol* **129**: 182–188.
13. Lanigan SW. (1996) Port wine stains on the lower limb: response to pulsed dye laser therapy. *Clin Exp Dermatol* **21**: 88–92.
14. Nguyen CM, Yohn JJ, Huff C, *et al.* (1998) Facial port wine stains in childhood: prediction of the rate of improvement as a function of the age of the patient, size and location of the port wine stain and the number of treatments with the pulsed dye (585 nm) laser. *Br J Dermatol* **138**: 821–825.
15. Goh CL. (2000) Flashlamp-pumped pulsed dye laser (585 nm) for the treatment of portwine stains — a study of treatment outcome in 94 Asian patients in Singapore. *Singapore Med J* **41**: 24–28.
16. Yang MU, Yaroslavsky AN, Farinelli WA, *et al.* (2005) Long-pulsed neodymium: yttrium-aluminum-garnet laser treatment for port-wine stains. *J Am Acad Dermatol* **52**: 480–490.
17. Izikson L, Nelson JS, Anderson RR. (2009) Treatment of hypertrophic and resistant port wine stains with a 755 nm laser: a case series of 20 patients. *Lasers Surg Med* **41**: 427–432.
18. Ho WS, Ying SY, Chan PC, *et al.* (2004) Treatment of port wine stains with intense pulsed light: a prospective study. *Dermatol Surg* **30**: 887–890.
19. Bjerring P, Christiansen K, Troilius A. (2003) Intense pulsed light source for the treatment of dye laser resistant port-wine stains. *J Cosmet Laser Ther* **5**: 7–13.
20. Bruckner AL, Frieden IJ. (2003) Hemangiomas of infancy. *J Am Acad Dermatol* **48**: 477–493.
21. Cantatore JL, Kriegel DA. (2004) Laser surgery: an approach to the pediatric patient. *J Am Acad Dermatol* **50**: 165–184.
22. Batta K, Goodyear HM, Moss C, *et al.* (2002) Randomised controlled study of early pulsed dye laser treatment of uncomplicated childhood haemangiomas: results of a 1-year analysis. *Lancet* **360**: 521–527.
23. Tay YK, Weston WL, Morelli JG. (1997) Treatment of pyogenic granuloma in children with the flashlamp-pumped pulsed dye laser. *Pediatrics* **99**: 368–370.
24. Omura NE, Dover JS, Arndt KA, *et al.* (2003) Treatment of reticular leg veins with a 1064 nm long-pulsed Nd:YAG laser. *J Am Acad Dermatol* **48**: 76–81.
25. Baumler W, Ulrich H, Hartl A, *et al.* (2006) Optimal parameters for the treatment of leg veins using Nd:YAG lasers at 1064 nm. *Br J Dermatol* **155**: 364–371.
26. Varma S, Lanigan SW. (2000) Laser therapy of telangiectatic leg veins: clinical evaluation of the 810 nm diode laser. *Clin Exp Dermatol* **25**: 419–422.
27. Woo WK, Jasim ZF, Handley JM. (2003) 532 nm Nd: YAG and 595-nm pulsed dye laser treatment of leg telangiectasia using ultralong pulse duration. *Dermatol Surg* **29**: 1176–1180.
28. Park HS, Choi WS. (2008) Pulsed dye laser treatment for viral warts: a study of 120 patients. *J Dermatol* **35**: 491–498.
29. Sethuraman G, Richards KA, Hiremagalore RN, *et al.* (2010) Effectiveness of pulsed dye laser in the treatment of recalcitrant warts in children. *Dermatol Surg* **36**: 58–65.
30. Manuskiatti W, Wanitphakdeedecha R, Fitzpatrick RE. (2007) Effect of pulse width of a 595 nm flashlamp-pumped pulsed dye laser on the treatment response of keloidal and hypertrophic sternotomy scars. *Dermatol Surg* **33**: 152–161.

Chapter 5

Treatment of Pigmented Lesions in the Asian Skin

Yong-Kwang Tay*

Introduction

Asian skin, Fitzpatrick's skin phototypes III–VI, differs from Caucasian skin, phototypes I–II, in several aspects (Table 5.1). Firstly, Asian skin is more pigmented, due to the presence of more epidermal melanin compared to the lighter Caucasian skin. This is because of the larger melanosomes and the higher level of melanin production in the darker skin types.[1] Due to the higher epidermal melanin content of ethnic skin, there is an increased risk of post-inflammatory hyperpigmentation following the use of light sources and lasers.

Secondly, the main manifestation of photoaging in Asians is pigmentary changes, such as solar lentigines, seborrheic keratoses, Hori's nevus, and melasma, which often coexist, rather than wrinkling. Skin wrinkling in the ethnic people of South East Asia is not apparent until the age of about 50 years and the degree of wrinkling is not as marked as in Caucasian skin.[2]

Thirdly, conditions like rosacea, especially the erythematous telangiectatic variant, are less common in the Asian skin compared to white skin. For all laser procedures, sun protection with advice to avoid excessive sun exposure, to use umbrellas, the consistent use of a broad-spectrum sunscreen (sun protection factor ≥30), and a topical bleaching regimen should be instituted at least 2–3 months before the procedure and restarted as soon as possible postoperatively, when the skin has healed. This is important to reduce the risk of post-inflammatory hyperpigmentation and to prevent recurrence.

Several bleaching agents, e.g. hydroquinone, tretinoin, glycolic acid, azelaic acid, vitamin C, and kojic acid, have been used, usually in combination. Hydroquinone suppresses new melanogenesis by inhibiting the conversion of dopa to melanin via enzymatic inhibition of tyrosinase. Tretinoin improves pigmentation by accelerating the discharge of epidermal melanin through desquamation. The combination of hydroquinone and tretinoin is an effective method for the removal of epidermal pigmentation.[3] In the author's practice, all patients are given a combination of 4% hydroquinone cream twice a day, ascorbic acid cream in the morning, tretinoin 0.025–0.05% cream at night and sunscreen daily. Ascorbic acid cream helps to lighten pigmentation by suppressing melanin synthesis through its antioxidant effect and is usually well tolerated with very few side effects.[4]

Pigment-specific Lasers

Various laser systems can be used to remove pigmented lesions. Melanin is the main chromophore and melanosomes, the organelle in which melanin is stored, are the primary target of laser-induced damage.[5] Melanin has a broad absorption spectrum, from ultraviolet range through the visible and infrared

*Chief and Senior Consultant, Department of Dermatology, Changi General Hospital, Singapore.

Table 5.1.

Fitzpatrick Classification of Skin Type

I.	Always burns, never tans
II.	Burns easily, tans minimally
III.	Burns moderately, tans moderately
IV.	Burns minimally, tans moderately
V.	Rarely burns, tans profusely
VI.	Never burns, tans profusely

Table 5.2.

Q-switched Lasers

Wavelength (nm)	Laser	Indication*
532 (green)	Fd Nd:YAG	Epidermal pigmented lesions
694 (red)	Ruby	Epidermal and dermal pigmented lesions
755 (infrared)	Alexandrite	Epidermal and dermal pigmented lesions
1064 (infrared)	Nd:YAG	Dermal pigmented lesions

*Epidermal pigmented lesions: e.g. ephelides, lentigines, café-au-lait macules, nevus spilus. Mixed pigmented lesions (epidermal and dermal component): e.g. Becker's nevus, melasma: Dermal pigmented lesions, e.g. nevus of Ota, nevus of Ito, Hori's nevus, congenital nevus.

spectra. A selective window for targeting melanin lies between 600 and 1100 nm, where there is good skin penetration and greater absorption of melanin over oxyhemoglobin.[6] The most widely used pigment-specific lasers are the Quality (Q)-switched lasers. The effect of Q-switching allows the delivery of powerful laser pulses with high peak power within a very short pulse duration of a few nanoseconds. The thermal relaxation time (the time needed for an object to cool to one-half of its original temperature) of a melanosome is about 0.5–1 microsecond (μs).[5] According to the theory of selective photothermolysis,[7] the pulse duration must be less than the thermal relaxation time of the target to cause preferential confined injury to the chromophore. The Q-switched lasers, with their nanosecond pulse duration, can selectively target melanosomes and tattoo particles.

The Q-switched (QS) lasers in use today are the Q-switched ruby laser (694 nm, 25–40 nanoseconds), the Q-switched alexandrite laser (755 nm, 50–100 nanoseconds), and the Q-switched neodymium: yttrium–aluminum-garnet (Nd:YAG) laser (1064 nm, 5–10 nanoseconds[8] (Table 5.2). By placing a frequency doubling (Fd) potassium-titanyl-phosphate (KTP) crystal, the 1064 nm wavelength may be halved to 532 nm (green light).

Whatever laser system is used, treatment should be initiated at the threshold fluence (i.e. the minimum fluence producing immediate tissue whitening). This whitening (clinical endpoint) may be due to nitrogen bubble formation from the photomechanical effects of Q-switched laser pulses resulting in rapid expansion, cavitation, and rupture of the melanosomes.[7] This whitening fades within a few minutes due to the dissolution of the gas bubbles. This is followed by erythema, edema, and (at higher fluences) punctuate bleeding. These petechiae may represent indirect vascular injury, resulting from the pressure waves generated by the laser on the dermal melanocytes around the blood vessels.[9]

Patients with darker skin types require longer wavelengths as in the 1064 nm Nd:YAG, as there is less absorption by epidermal melanin at this wavelength, resulting in a lower risk of epidermal injury and pigmentary alterations. In general, darker skin has a lower threshold dose for clinical whitening due to the higher epidermal melanin content.[10]

The use of long-pulsed (millisecond, or ms) pigment lasers in the treatment of lentigines and congenital nevi will be discussed under the individual sections.

Anesthesia and Postoperative Care

Topical anesthetic cream, e.g. EMLA®, a eutectic mixture of lidocaine 2.5% and prilocaine 2.5% within an oil-in-water emulsion, is applied under occlusion one hour before the procedure. General anesthesia may be rarely required, e.g. in the laser irradiation of extensive nevus of Ota or congenital nevus in young children. Eyes are protected with eye shields. Postoperative care consists of intermittent ice compression for 20 minutes after the procedure to reduce pain and swelling, normal saline washes, and application of aloe vera gel, until all crusts have flaked off. Sunscreen and topical bleaching agents should be restarted once healing is complete, usually within 1–2 weeks of treatment. It is advisable to take photographs before starting treatment and periodically after a few laser sessions to assess progress.

Epidermal Pigmented Lesions

Ephelides (Freckles)

Freckles are brown macules occurring on sun-exposed skin that darken following sun exposure. They appear in childhood and increase during the summer. Frequency decreases with age. On histology, ephelides are characterized by hyperpigmentation of the basal layer without elongation of the rete ridges and with no increase in the number of epidermal melanocytes.[11] These lesions respond well to the QS ruby,[12] QS alexandrite,[13] and QS Fd Nd:YAG (532 nm)[14] lasers after one or two treatments. Re-exposure without adequate sun protection stimulates new freckle recurrence.

Case 1

A 14-year-old Chinese girl had presented with numerous ephelides since the age of eight years. The lesions were treated with the QS 532 nm Nd:YAG laser using a 3 mm spot size, fluence of 1.2 J/cm^2, and a repetition rate of 5 Hz. The freckles were cleared after one treatment (Fig. 5.1).

Lentigines

Lentigines are common brown, circumscribed macules, increasing in number with age and occurring on the chronic sun-exposed skin of the face, forearms, and hands. On histology, solar lentigines have elongated and clubbed rete ridges and the basal cell layer

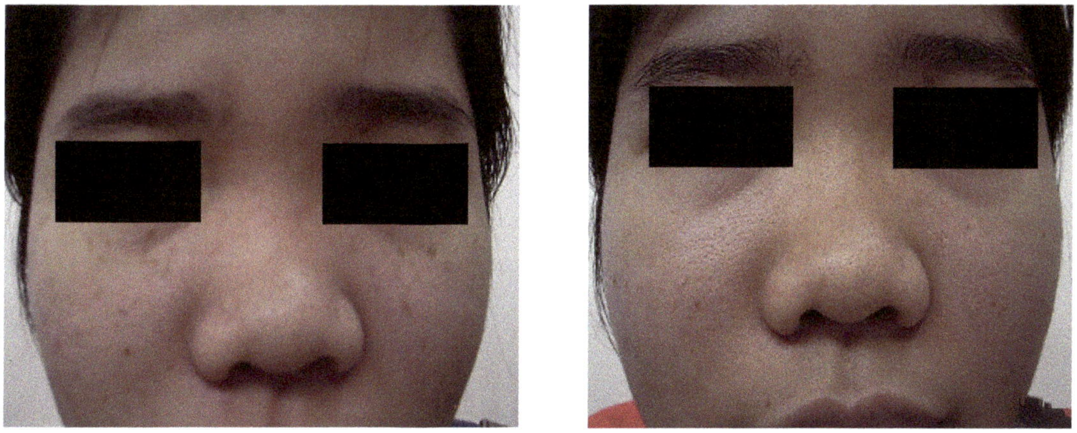

(a) (b)

Figure 5.1.

Case 1. Ephelides. (a) Before treatment. (b) After (QS 532 nm Nd:YAG laser).

shows hypermelanosis with an increase in the number of melanocytes.[11] Lentigines can also be part of a syndrome, e.g. Peutz-Jeghers syndrome, Laugier-Hunziker syndrome, etc., and can occur in otherwise healthy people on the lower lips.

All the Q-switched lasers are highly effective in clearing lentigines, usually in one or two treatment sessions. In the author's practice, treatment intervals range from 4–6 months to allow any post-inflammatory hyperpigmentation that may develop to subside before embarking on another treatment. Sadighha *et al.* treated 91 patients with solar lentigines (skin types II–IV) with the Q-switched ruby laser (3 mm spot, fluence 8–16 J/cm^2) and noted complete clearance in all patients after one to two treatment sessions.[15] Post-inflammatory hyperpigmentation occurred in 7.8% of patients in skin type II, 9.8% in skin type III, and 16.6% in skin type IV. Hypopigmentation was seen in one patient and all pigmentary changes improved over six months.

Tse *et al.* compared the use of the Q-switched ruby laser (5 mm spot, fluence 7 J/cm^2) with the 532 nm Q-switched Nd:YAG laser (3 mm spot, 2.4 J/cm^2) and noted 67% clearing with the ruby laser vs 58% clearing with the 532 nm Nd:YAG laser, suggesting that the ruby laser was more effective.[16] Suh *et al.* treated 12 patients with lentigines with the 532 nm Q-switched Nd:YAG laser (3 mm spot, fluence 1.1–4.4 J/cm^2, repetition rate 10 Hz) and noted good to excellent responses in 10 patients with two treatments at 3-monthly intervals.[14] Wang *et al.* treated 17 patients with lentigines with one session of the Q-switched alexandrite laser (3 mm spot, 6.5–7.5 J/cm^2) and noted a 61% improvement rate at three months.[13] However, in 47% of patients, post-inflammatory hyper-pigmentation developed that resolved within six months.

Case 2

A 45-year-old Chinese woman presented with facial lentigines of four years duration. The lesions were treated with the QS 532 nm Nd:YAG laser using a 3 mm spot size and fluence of 1.4 J/cm^2. Significant clearing of the lentigines were noted two months after one treatment (Fig. 5.2).

Labial lentigines (labial melanotic macules), occurring either as part of Laugier-Hunziker syndrome, Peutz-Jeghers syndrome, or in healthy individuals, respond uniformly well to the Q-switched lasers (Fig. 5.3). Usually, one or two treatments are needed to clear with no recurrences after one to two years of followup.[17–20] Treatment is well tolerated, with

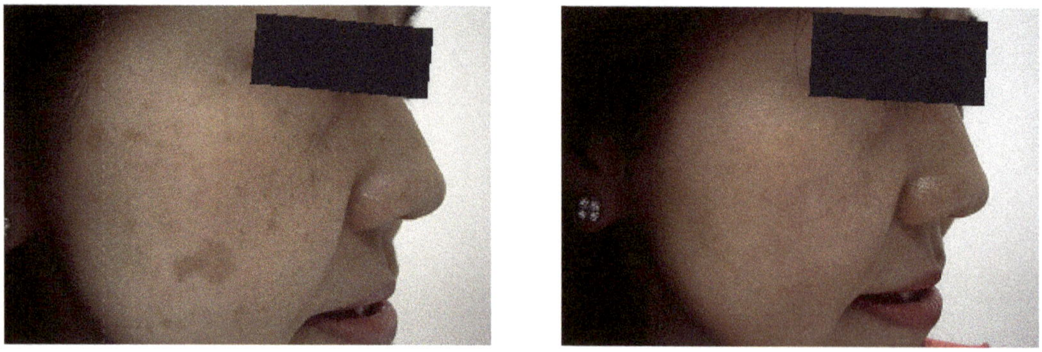

(a) (b)

Figure 5.2.

Case 2. Lentigines. (a) Before treatment. (b) After (QS 532 nm Nd:YAG laser).

erythema and edema occurring immediately after laser irradiation and crusting after two days, sloughing off within a week.[20] Although lesions may recur, they can be retreated without loss of efficacy.[19]

The risk of postinflammatory hyperpigmentation (PIH) after the use of the Q-switched lasers for the treatment of ephelides and lentigines ranges from about 17%[15] to 28%[13] in ethnic skin. The mechanism of this PIH may be due to the induction by the Q-switched laser beams of melanogenic stimulatory cytokines such as basic fibroblast growth factor, hepatocyte growth factor, and stem cell factor in fibroblasts.[21] Another possible mechanism is the photomechanical effects of Q-switched lasers causing damage and inflammation of the superficial blood vessels, resulting in PIH.[22]

The use of long-pulsed lasers and intense pulsed light (IPL) devices have been shown to reduce the risk of PIH.[13,23–27] Chan *et al.* showed that the 532 nm long-pulsed Nd:YAG laser (2 mm spot, fluence 9–12 J/cm^2, 2 ms pulse duration, ashen-gray appearance as the clinical endpoint) had a similar degree of clearing compared with the Q-switched 532 nm Nd:YAG laser (2 mm spot, fluence 1 J/cm^2) in the treatment of facial lentigines but a lower risk of PIH.[23] To reduce the risk of scarring, the chosen pulse duration should be shorter than the thermal relaxation time of the epidermis, which is estimated to be about 10 ms.

Rashid *et al.* treated 20 patients (skin type IV) with freckles and lentigines with a quasi-continuous Nd:YAG (532 nm) laser 3–8 times, at 4–12 weekly intervals, and noted that 16 patients had more than 50% improvement.[24] Side effects included hypo-pigmentation (25%), textural changes (15%), and hyperpigmentation (10%), but these were mild and resolved within six months. Rosenbach *et al.* treated 21 patients with solar lentigines two times with an alexandrite laser (7 mm spot, fluence 35–40 J/cm^2, 5 ms pulse duration) and noted excellent improvement in 19 patients.[25] Treatment interval was four weeks and the clinical endpoint was perilesional erythema and edema. There was no PIH, but 2 treated lesions developed mild hypopigmentation.

Trafeli *et al.* treated 18 patients with solar lentigines once with a long-pulsed alexandrite laser and noted that shorter pulse widths and treatment without cryogen cooling lowered the threshold fluence for clearance.[26] Darker lentigines had greater clearance compared with lighter-colored ones and there was no PIH.

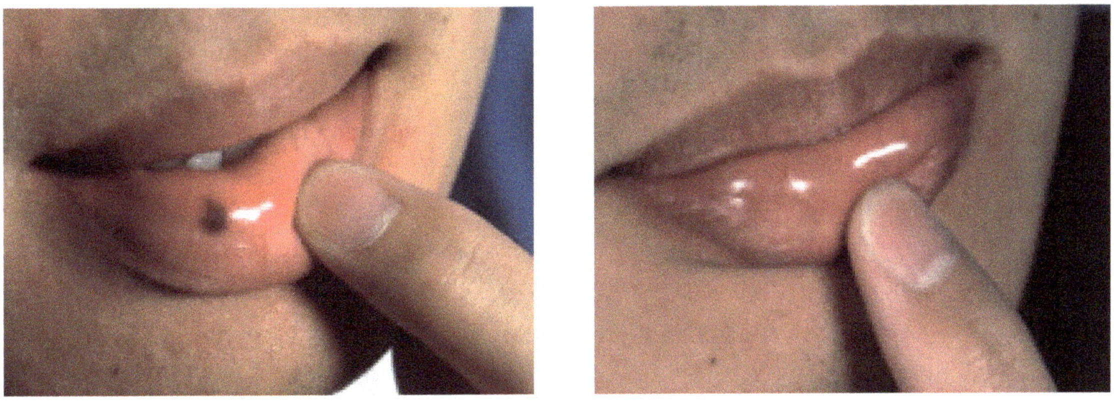

(a) (b)

Figure 5.3.

Case 3. Labial melanotic macule. (a) Before treatment. (b) After one treatment showing complete clearance. (QS 532 nm Nd:YAG: 3 mm spot, 1.4 J/cm^2.)

Kono *et al.* compared the Q-switched ruby laser (4 mm spot, fluence 6–7 J/cm^2) with the long-pulsed dye laser with compression (595 nm, 7 mm spot, fluence 10–13 J/cm^2, pulse duration 1.5 ms, no cryogen cooling, ash-gray color change as the clinical endpoint) for the treatment of facial lentigines in 18 Asian patients.[27] Compression of the skin by a glass window attached to the tip of the handpiece removed blood from the cutaneous vessels and this removed absorption by hemoglobin and allowed the long-pulsed dye laser to treat lentigines without purpura. The degree of clearing of the lentigines after one treatment was 70% for the Q-switched ruby laser and 83% for the long-pulsed dye laser. PIH was seen in four patients after Q-switched ruby laser, but none after long-pulsed dye laser.

From these studies, it is clear that the long-pulsed lasers are effective and safe in the treatment of ephelides and lentigines with a lower risk of PIH, but these long-pulsed systems may require more treatment sessions, e.g. 3–5, to produce lesion clearance compared to Q-switched lasers.[13,24]

Café-au-lait macules

Café-au-lait macules (CALMs) are well-circumscribed brown macules and patches that may occur as isolated lesions or associated with neurocutaneous syndromes like neurofibromatosis or McCune-Albright syndrome. They appear at birth and may increase in number with age and are persistent. On histology there is melanocytic hyperplasia present in the basal layer of the epidermis. Macromelanosomes are present in the CALMs only in patients with neurofibromatosis.[28]

A variety of lasers have been tried on CALMs with variable results. Any of the Q-switched lasers may be used, including the Q-switched 532 nm Nd:YAG laser,[14,16,28] the Q-switched ruby laser,[16,28] and the Q-switched alexandrite laser.[29] Other lasers that have been tried include the 510 nm pigmented dye laser,[30] copper vapor laser[31] and the erbium:YAG laser.[32] Recently, the 1064 nm Q-switched Nd:YAG laser (4 mm spot, fluence 2.5–2.8 J/cm^2, 2 passes) was used successfully to treat a segmental facial café-au-lait patch.[33] The patient underwent 10 treatments at 2-weekly intervals with distinct clearing.

Café-au-lait macules respond unpredictably to laser treatments. Multiple treatments at 3–4 monthly intervals are required for lightening and recurrences are common, seen in up to 50% of treated lesions.[34] Recurrence may occur as early as three months after initial clearance,[28] but are often responsive to further treatments. The mechanisms underlying the frequent recurrence of CALMs after laser therapy are unknown, but may involve a temporary disruption in the melanocyte-keratinocyte melanosome transfer mechanism followed by their gradual repopulation.[28] This variable response implies a subset of lesions with unique biologic behavior. Café-au-lait macules in association with neurofibromatosis do not respond as well to the Q-switched lasers compared to those CALMs without under-lying neurofibromatosis.[14] This may be due to the presence of macromelanosomes that are present in patients with neurofibromatosis. In the author's experience, facial CALMs and smaller lesions appear to be more responsive to treatment. Test spots are recommended prior to treating the entire lesion.

Case 4

A 17-year-old girl presented with a café-au-lait patch on the left cheek since birth. The lesion was treated twice at 4-month intervals with the QS 532 nm Nd:YAG laser using a 3 mm spot and a fluence of 1.5 J/cm^2 with long term resolution (Fig. 5.4).

Nevus spilus

Nevus spilus, or speckled lentiginous nevus, presents as darkly pigmented macules or papules scattered over a large brown patch. They can be considered as café-au-lait macules with focal hyperpigmentation, representing either junctional or compound nevi.[35]

Like café-au-lait macules, nevus spilus responds variably to laser treatment. Incomplete clearing or recurrences are fairly common, and test spots are recommended prior to treatment. Any of

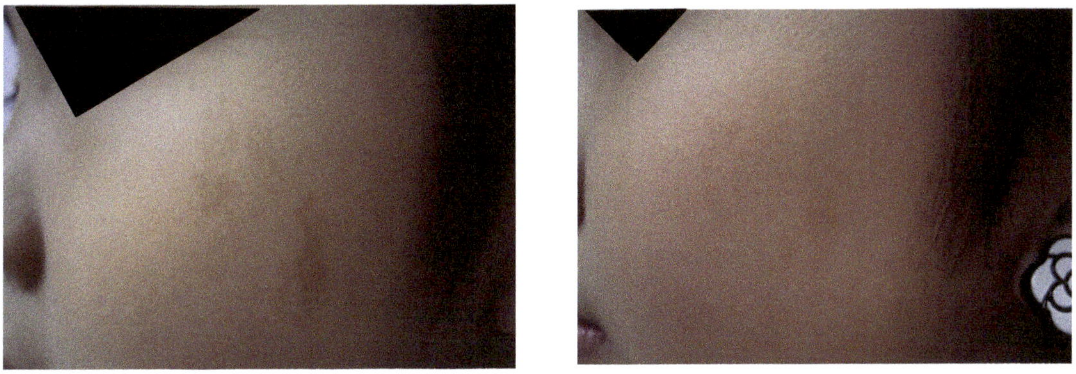

(a) (b)

Figure 5.4.

Case 4. Café-au-lait patch. (a) Before treatment. (b) After (QS 532 nm Nd:YAG laser).

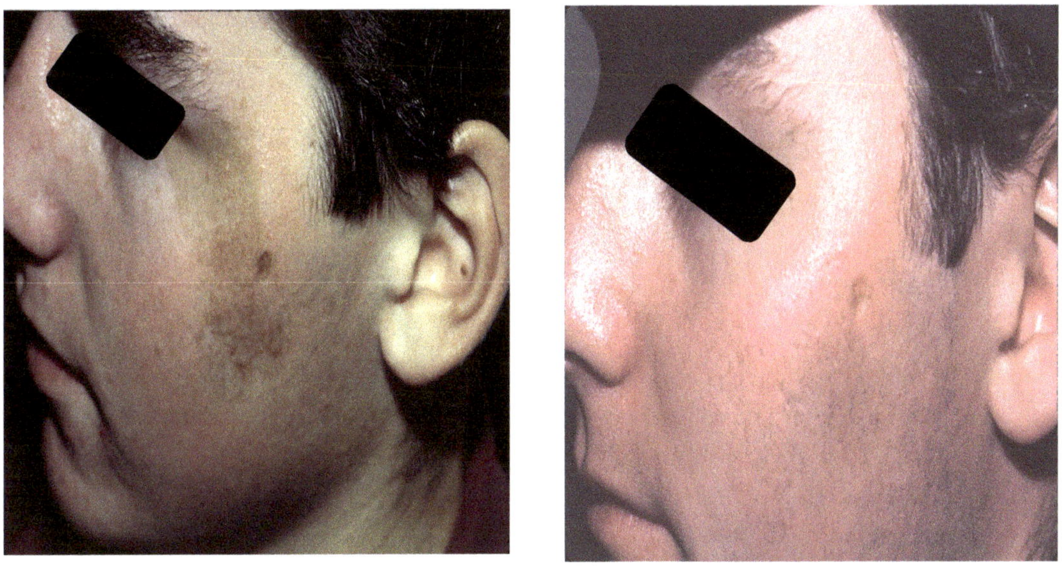

(a) (b)

Figure 5.5.

Case 5. Café-au-lait patch. (a) Before treatment. (b) After 5 treatments showing clearance: QS alexandrite laser: 3 mm spot, 7–9 J/cm^2. (Courtesy of Morelli JG, MD, Denver, USA.)

the Q-switched lasers may be used, including the Q-switched 532 nm Nd:YAG laser[14,16] (Fig. 5.6) the Q-switched ruby laser,[16,35,36] and the Q-switched alexandrite laser.[37] The Q-switched ruby laser (5 mm spot, fluence 5.5–8 J/cm^2) was more effective in removing pigment compared to the Q-switched 532 nm Nd:YAG laser (3 mm spot, fluence 3.4 J/cm^2) in the study by Grevelink.[35] Multiple treatments (2–5 or more at 2–3-monthly intervals) were required for improvement.[35,37] The junctional or compound component of nevus spilus is more easily removed compared to the café-au-lait component, which tends to be more resistant, requires more treatments, and may recur.[35,36]

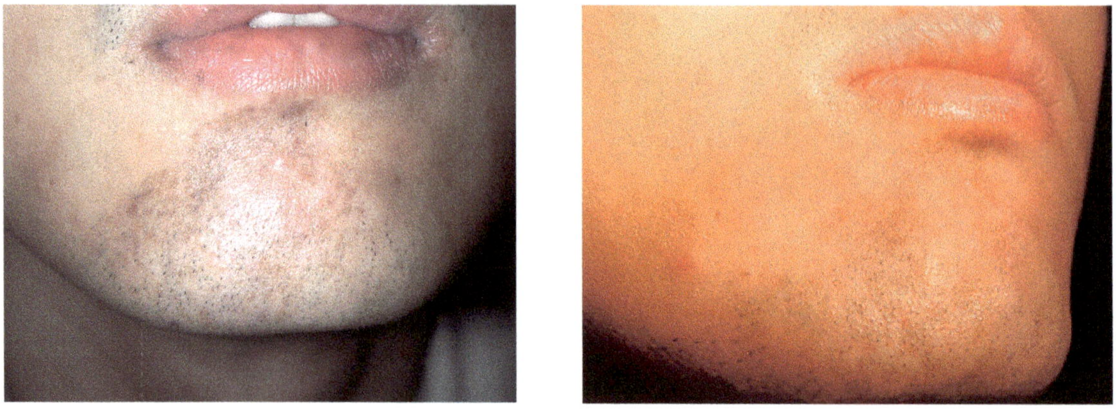

(a) (b)

Figure 5.6.

Case 6. Nevus spilus. (a) Before treatment. (b) After 5 treatments at 3–4 monthly intervals showing lightening. (QS 532 nm Nd:YAG laser: 3 mm spot, 3 J/cm^2.)

Mixed Epidermal-Dermal Pigmented Lesions

Becker's Nevus

Becker's nevus is a fairly common hamartoma characterized by brown pigmentation and hypertrichosis, occurring over the shoulder and back predominantly in young men, appearing during puberty.[38] Histologically, Becker's nevus shows mild hyperkeratosis, elongation of the rete ridges, and basal cell layer hyperpigmentation. The number of melanocytes is normal or slightly increased and the melanin content of the keratinocytes is high. Melanophages may be present in the papillary dermis in addition to hypertrophied sebaceous glands and bundles of smooth muscle fibers.

With the use of the Q-switched pigment lasers, complete clearing is rarely achieved and many sessions are necessary.[14,16,39] The Q-switched ruby laser appears to be more effective than the Q-switched 532 nm Nd:YAG laser.[16] Trellers *et al.* compared the use of the erbium:YAG laser (2940 nm, 3 mm spot, fluence 28 J/cm^2, one treatment) to the Q-switched Nd:YAG (1064 nm, 3 mm spot, fluence 10 J/cm^2, three treatments at 2-monthly intervals) in 22 patients with Becker's nevus.[39] The erbium:YAG laser was significantly more effective, with complete clearance in 6 of 11 patients compared with only 1 of 11 patients with the 1064 nm Nd:YAG laser at two years. Side effects included erythema, which lasted longer with the erbium:YAG laser (three months) vs 15 days with the Q-switched Nd:YAG laser, mild textural changes in three patients, and mild repigmentation in five patients. Hair density was not affected by the two laser systems.[39]

The long-pulsed ruby[40] and long-pulsed alexandrite laser[41] have been used to decrease pigmentation and hair density. Choi *et al.*[41] treated 11 Korean patients with Becker's nevus using the alexandrite laser (15–18 mm spot, fluence 20–25 J/cm^2, 3 ms pulse duration, no cryogen cooling). Cryogen cooling was not used so as to destroy the epidermal melanin. Seven patients had good to excellent responses after multiple treatments (2–12) at 2–3-monthly intervals. Improvement was maintained at one year follow-up. Side effects included mild textural change and hypopigmentation in some patients and a hypertrophic scar in one patient. In all patients, hair density was decreased. It is thought that the long-term pigment reduction that occurs with the long-pulsed lasers is due to damage of the melanocytes in the deep hair follicules.[41]

Fractional resurfacing using the 1550 nm erbium-doped fiber laser was recently introduced as a safe and effective new treatment modality for Becker's nevus. Multiple treatment sessions (5–6) resulted in a greater than 75% pigment reduction.[42] However, there was no improvement in the hypertrichosis with this modality.

Melasma

Melasma is a common acquired pigmentary disorder manifesting as symmetric brown or rayish-brown facial hypermelanosis. It is more commonly seen in women, especially those with darker complexions (Fitzpatrick's skin types IV–VI) such as in the Asian and Hispanic population. Common predisposing factors include genetic predilection, ultraviolet light exposure, pregnancy, use of hormonal preparations, and certain cosmetics and photoxic drugs.[43] Three clinical patterns of melasma are recognized: (i) centrofacial pattern (63%), which affects the forehead, cheeks, nose, upper lip, and chin; (ii) malar pattern (21%), localized to the malar region; and (iii) a mandibular pattern (16%), localized to the ramus of the mandible.[44] Histopathologically, melasma is characterized by epidermal hyperpigmentation due to an increased number and activity of melanocytes and to increased activity of melanogenic enzymes.[44,45] Examination under Wood's light is useful in localizing the pigment and this has therapeutic implications.[44] Epidermal melasma appears light brown clinically and, under Wood's light, the pigmentation is intensified (darkened). The dermal type appears bluish-gray clinically and will not show this accentuation under Wood's light. The mixed type of melasma involves a deposition of melanin in both epidermal and dermal locations and there is color enhancement in some areas but not in others under Wood's light.

Melasma is a challenging condition to manage because of its chronic and recurrent nature. The mainstays of therapy are sun protection with a broad-spectrum sunscreen, which must be continued indefinitely to minimize the reactivation of melanocytes, and a topical bleaching regimen supplemented by superficial chemical peels.[43,46,47] Topical bleaching agents include hydroquinone, tretinoin, glycolic acid, kojic acid, azelaic acid, ascorbic acid, and orticosteroids, often used in combination.[43,47] Whilethe epidermal component often responds to bleachingagents, the dermal pigmentation is generally resistant.[46]

Melasma responds variably to laser treatments, and the use of lasers should be reserved for patients with refractory melasma who do not respond to topical bleaching agents and chemical peels. Laser treatments should always be combined with sun avoidance, hydroquinone, tretinoin, and other bleaching agents, to reduce the risk of recurrence. The use of the Q-switched ruby laser has been reported to be ineffective in four women (skin types III–V) with refractory melasma.[9] Side effects included worsened hyperpigmentation, no change, and confetti-like hypopigmentation.

The efficacy of the Q-switched alexandrite laser[48] and the 1064 nm Q-switched Nd:YAG laser using low fluences[49,50] has been reported in melasma. Cho *et al.* treated 25 women (skin types IV) with moderate to severe melasma using the Q-switched 1064 nm Nd:YAG laser (6 mm spot, 2.5 J/cm^2, 2 passes) at 2-weekly intervals.[50] The number of treatments ranged from 5 to 15, with a mean of seven treatments. There was a near-total clearance in seven patients, 16 had a moderate to marked clinical improvement, and two had no improvement. Treatment was well tolerated with post-treatment erythema lasting for a few hours. Temporary post-treatment hypopigmentation was noted in two patients.[50] This punctuate leucodermais thought to be caused by phototoxic damage to the melanocytes and may be persistent.[51] The punctuate leucoderma may be prevented by spacing out the treatment intervals to allow time for the melanocytes to recover.

Case 7

A 50-year-old woman presented with mixed type of melasma that was persistent and had minimal improvement with topical bleaching agents (Fig. 5.7). She underwent 5 Q-switched 1064 nm laser treatments at 2–3 monthly intervals using a 6 mm spot and a fluence of 2.5–3 J/cm^2, with a clinical endpoint of mild erythema.

The clinical endpoint should be mild erythema when lasers or intense pulsed light (IPL) devices are used to treat melasma, so as to avoid excessive thermal injury that can increase the risk of post-laser darkening.[22]

Resurfacing lasers, either alone or combined with a pigment-specific laser, may be useful for the treatment of refractory melasma. The aim of the ablative laser is to remove the superficial part of the skin, including the abnormal melanocytes. Patients with refractory melasma were treated once with the 2940 nm erbium:YAG laser and, despite marked improvement immediately after treatment, all patients developed PIH 3–6 weeks postoperatively.[52] The PIH resolved with glycolic acid peels, azelaic acid cream, and sunscreens and, at the end of six months, significant improvement in the melasma was noted.

In another study, a low-fluence, short-pulsed erbium:YAG laser was used to treat 20 Thai women with epidermal melasma (7 mm spot, fluence of 160 mJ [0.4 J/cm^2] and pulse duration of 300 μs).[53] Two treatments were given at monthly intervals. Treatment was well tolerated, with erythema lasting for 24 hours and complete re-epithelialization in 4–5 days. Three patients developed PIH. At the 4-month follow-up, about half the patients had moderate to excellent improvement, but 27% of patients showed no improvement, and recurrence of melasma occurred three months after discontinuation of treatment, suggesting the importance of concomitant bleaching agents and sunscreen to maintain the improvement.

Complete resolution of dermal melasma was noted after treatment with both pulsed CO_2 laser alone or pulsed CO_2 laser followed by the Q-switched alexandrite laser.[54] Two patients in the CO_2 laser-only group developed peripheral PIH. The CO_2 laser removes the hyperpigmentation in the epidermis by removing the epidermis and the denuded dermis can then be treated with the Q-switched alexandrite laser, which targets dermal melanin. A split-face study of six Thai women found that one pass of a CO_2 laser followed by one pass of the Q-switched alexandrite laser was more effective than one pass of the Q-switched alexandrite laser alone in the treatment of refractory melasma.[55]

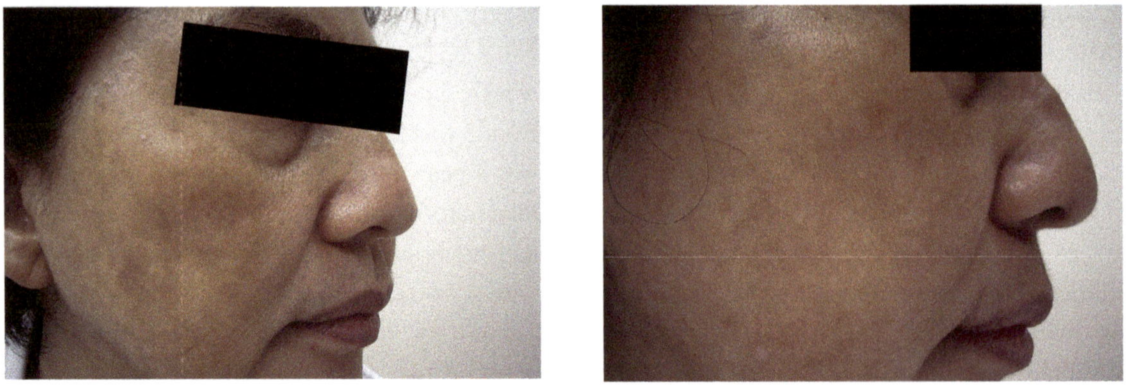

(a) (b)

Figure 5.7.

Case 7. Mixed melasma. (a) Before treatment. (b) After 5 treatments showing a moderate improvement in the melasma.

Three cases developed PIH on both sides that was effectively treated with bleaching agents. Transient hypopigmentation and contact dermatitis was seen in one patient with the combination treatment.

Fractional photothermolysis has recently been evaluated in the treatment of melasma, with encouraging results.[56–59] Rokhsar *et al.*[57] treated 10 women with melasma using the Fraxel laser™ (Reliant Technologies) with the following parameters: 1550 nm wavelength, fluence of 6–12 mJ per microthermal zone (MTZ) for a total of 2000–3500 MTZ/cm^2. Four to six treatment sessions were performed at 1–2 week intervals. Sixty percent of patients achieved 75–100% clearance. However, 30% had less than 25% improvement, and one patient developed PIH.

Lee *et al.*[59] treated 25 patients with melasma using the 1550 nm erbium-doped fractional photothermolysis laser at a fluence of 15 mJ/MTZ and a density of 125 MTZ/pass with eight passes. Four treatment sessions were performed at monthly intervals. At four weeks after the final treatment, 60% of patients had clinical improvement, but this decreased to 52% at 24 weeks after treatment. Ten patients (40%) had no change in the melasma at four weeks after the final treatment session. PIH was observed in three patients. A possible mechanism for the improvement of melasma after fractional photothermolysis is the observation that some dermal material such as melanin is incorporated into the micro-epidermal necrotic debris and shuttled up the epidermis to be exfoliated through the stratum corneum.[60] Light and electron microscopy on post-treatment specimens show fewer melanocytes and a relative absence of melanin in the surrounding keratinocytes compared to pre-treatment specimens.[61]

Taken together, these studies show that melasma responds variably and unpredictably to laser therapy. Given the fairly high risk of PIH and its tendency to recur, in the author's opinion laser treatment should be considered only for medically recalcitrant melasma.

Dermal Pigmented Lesions

Nevus of Ota

Nevus of Ota is a dermal melanocytosis, common in the Asian population and characterized by a unilateral blue or gray-brown patch in the skin innervated by the first and second branches of the trigeminal nerve. Involvement of the sclera on the ipsilateral side is common and ophthalmologic evaluation for possible glaucoma is necessary in patients with ocular involvement.[62] The lesions are benign, although rare cases of malignant melanoma arising within a nevus of Ota have been reported, especially in white patients.[63] The lesion is present at birth in about half the cases, while the remainder usually appear by the second decade of life, especially around puberty. The condition is more common in women (4:1).[64] On histology, spindle-shaped dendritic melanocytes are scattered among collagen bundles in the papillary and reticular dermis. Nevus of Ito has a similar clinical and histologic appearance to nevus of Ota but is found in the distribution of the posterior and lateral supraclavicular and lateral brachial cutaneous nerves over the scapular, supraclavicular, and deltoid areas.[65]

The Q-switched ruby,[66,67] the Q-switched alexandrite,[64,68,69] (Fig. 5.8) and the Q-switched 1064 nm Nd:YAG[70,71] (Figs. 5.9, 5.10) lasers provide an extremely effective and safe means of treating nevus of Ota. The degree of lightening is directly proportional to the number of treatments performed: the more treatments given, the better the results.[64,69] Higher energy fluences result in a greater degree of lightening compared to lower fluences,[67] and the response to laser treatment also depends on the color of the nevus. Using the Q-switched ruby laser, Ueda *et al.* showed that brown and violet lesions achieve optimal clearing after 3–4 laser treatments, in contrast to the more heavily pigmented blue-green nevi, which required six or more treatments to achieve the same degree of lightening.[72]

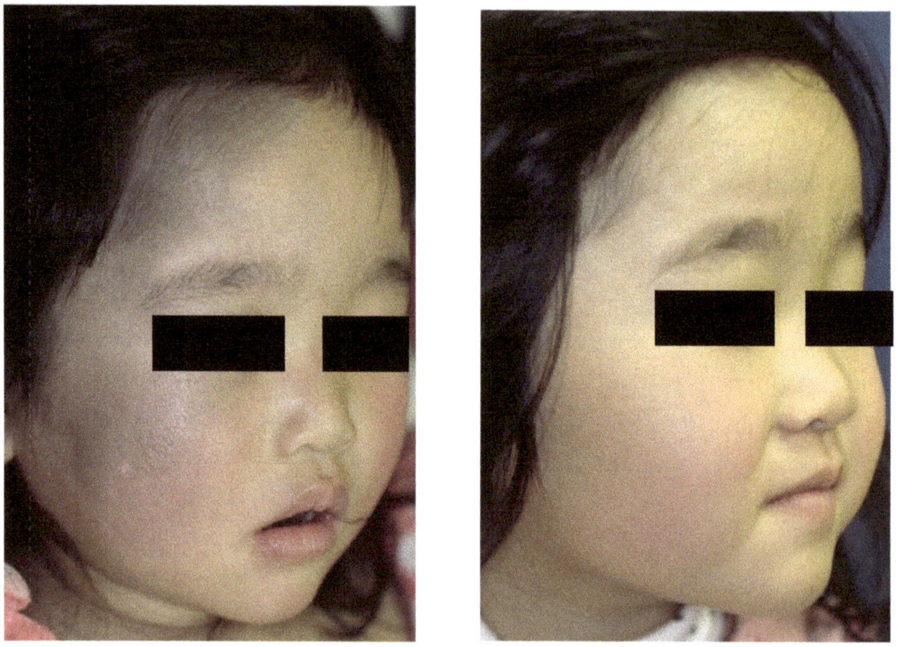

(a) (b)

Figure 5.8.

Case 8. Nevus of Ota. (a) Before treatment. (b) After 4 treatments with the QS alexandrite laser: 3 mm spot, 5–5.5 J/cm^2 at 3-monthly intervals. (Courtesy of Taro Kono, MD, PhD, Tokyo, Japan.)

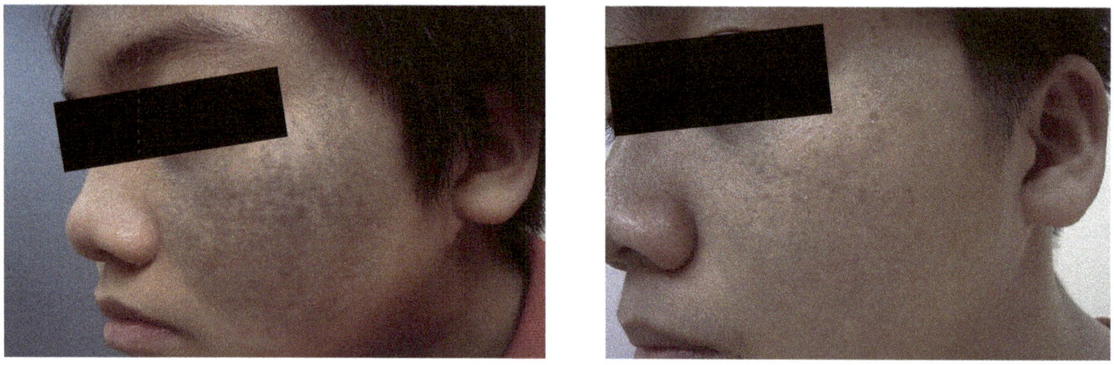

(a) (b)

Figure 5.9.

Case 9. Nevus of Ota. (a) Before treatment. (b) After 8 treatments with the QS 1064 nm Nd:YAG laser: 4 mm spot, 8 J/cm^2.

Using the Q-switched ruby laser (4 mm spot, 5–7 J/cm^2) at 3–4 monthly intervals, Kono *et al.*, showed that children with nevus of Ota require fewer sessions to achieve an excellent response compared to older age groups.[73] This advantage must be weighed against the risk of recurrence[74] and the need for multiple treatment sessions, possibly under general anesthesia, in children. In a study of 171 patients with nevus of Ota treated with the Q-switched alexandrite and Q-switched Nd:YAG lasers, 13 patients (7.6%) had recurrence of the nevus (mean time of recurrence was 39 months) after complete or near-complete clearance with laser treatment.[75]

The optimal interval between treatment sessions remains to be elucidated and many authorities wait for 3–4 months between sessions, although Zhong *et al.* suggested a treatment interval of 20–27 weeks as being optimal to allow time for the degenerated mela-nosomes to be scavenged and cleared by macr-ophages.[69] The Q-switched 1064 nm Nd:YAG laser (2 mm spot, 7–9 J/cm^2) appears to be more effective than the Q-switched alexandrite laser (2 mm spot, 6–9 J/cm^2) in lightening nevus of Ota. This may be due to the propensity of the Q-switched 1064 nm Nd:YAG laser to cause more blood and tissue splatter compared to the Q-switched alexandrite laser.[71] This may facilitate further lightening by means of transepidermal elimination. A higher rate of complications like hypo- and hyperpigmentation and textural change is seen with the Q-switched alexandrite laser compared to the Q-switched 1064 nm Nd:YAG laser, as the shorter 755 nm wavelength of the alexandrite laser is better absorbed by melanin and this causes more injury to the epidermal melanocytes in the darker Asian skin.[75] Recently, fractional photothermolysis using a fractionated 1440 nm Nd:YAG laser was successfully used to treat a patient with nevus of Ota resistant to the standard Q-switched 1064 nm Nd:YAG laser.[76]

Hori's Nevus

Hori's nevus, also known as acquired, bilateral nevus of Ota-like macules (ABNOM), an acquired

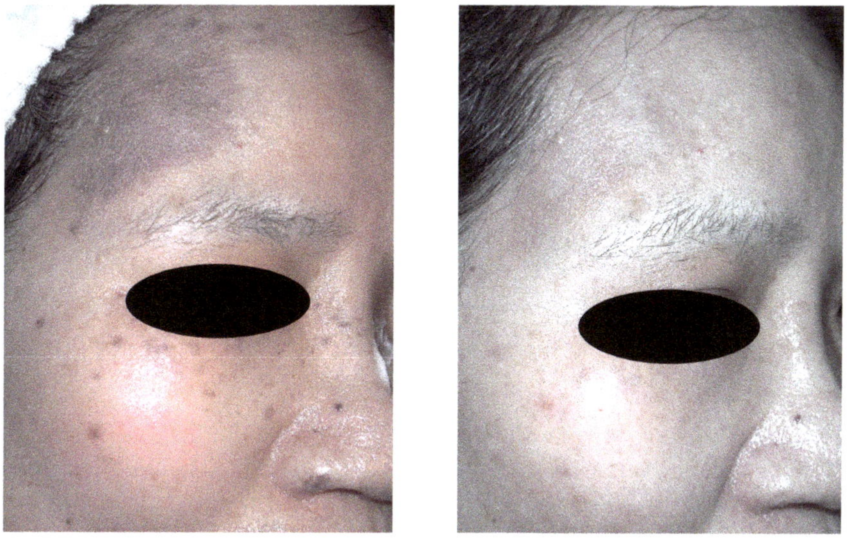

(a) (b)

Figure 5.10.

Case 10. Nevus of Ota. (a) Before treatment. (b) After 6 treatments with the QS 1064 nm Nd:YAG laser: 3 mm spot, 10 J/cm^2. (Courtesy of Lee GS, MD, Seoul, Korea.)

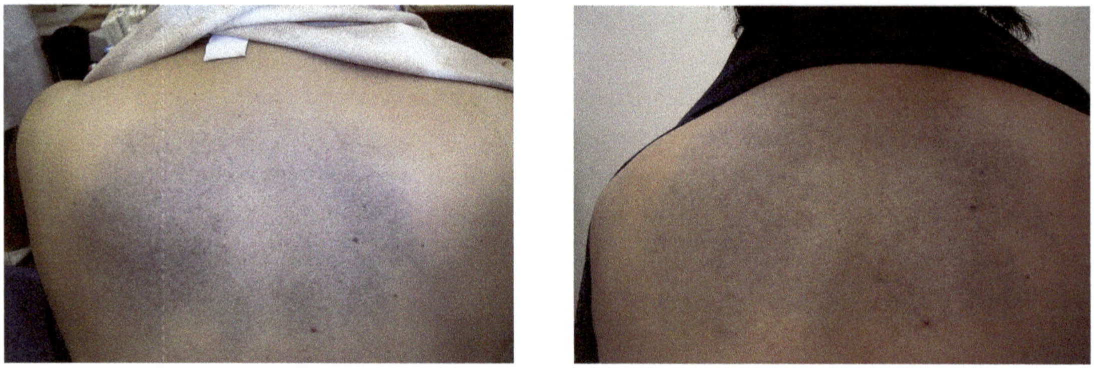

(a) (b)

Figure 5.11.

Case 11. Nevus of Ito. (a) Before treatment. (b) After 8 treatments with the QS 1064 nm Nd:YAG laser: 3 mm spot, 11 J/cm^2.

dermal melanocytosis, is characterized by multiple speckled blue-brown and/or slate-gray macules occurring bilaterally on the malar regions.[77] Less commonly, the temple, nose, forehead, and eyelids are affected. Early lesions consist of discrete brown macules, whereas confluent slate-gray macules become more common over time.[78] Hori's nevus is common in Asian women and usually presents after the third decade of life. Predisposing factors include chronic sun exposure, pregnancy, hormonal medication, and genetic influence.[78]

Hori's nevus can be distinguished clinically from nevus of Ota by its speckled and bilateral distribution, late onset in adulthood, and lack of mucosal involvement.[79] Histologically, in ABNOM, elongated spindle-shaped melanocytes are dispersed between the collagen fibers and perivascularly in the upper dermis. In contrast, melanocytes in nevus of Ota are distributed diffusely throughout the papillary and reticular dermis.[80]

The Q-switched ruby,[81] the Q-switched alexandrite,[80,82] and the Q-switched 1064 nm Nd:YAG[83–85] (Figs. 5.12, 5.13) lasers have all been used successfully for the treatment of Hori's nevus. The degree of lightening is proportional to the number of treatments performed: the more treatments given, the better the results.[82,84,85] Typical parameters for the treatment of Hori's nevus using the Q-switched ruby laser[81] are 2–5 mm spot and fluence of 7–10 J/cm^2; for the Q-switched alexandrite laser,[80,82] 3 mm spot, 7.5–8 J/cm^2; and for the Q-switched 1064 nm Nd:YAG laser,[85] 3 mm spot, 4.2–9.9 J/cm^2 (mean 7.8 J/cm^2). The treatment endpoint was immediate whitening and treatment intervals range from two weeks to six months.[81–85]

Hori's nevus is known to be more resistant to laser treatment, requiring more sessions compared to nevus of Ota. One of the reasons for this is the higher rate of PIH seen after laser treatments for Hori's nevus.[80,86] The incidence of PIH ranged from 7–73% of cases and was transient, fading in 2–6 months with 4% hydroquinone cream.[81,84] The high rate of PIH may be related to the greater clustering of melanocytes around the blood vessels, as indirect vessel injury from the laser treatment leads to a higher degree of erythema and subsequently PIH.[80] Post-inflammatory hypopigmentation, which may be permanent, is more commonly seen with the shorter wavelength ruby and alexandrite lasers and also if the sessions are not adequately spaced.[81,82]

In Hori's nevus, there is significant epidermal pigmentation. Methods to remove this epidermal pigmentation, thereby allowing more dermal penetration and greater efficacy, have been advocated. The

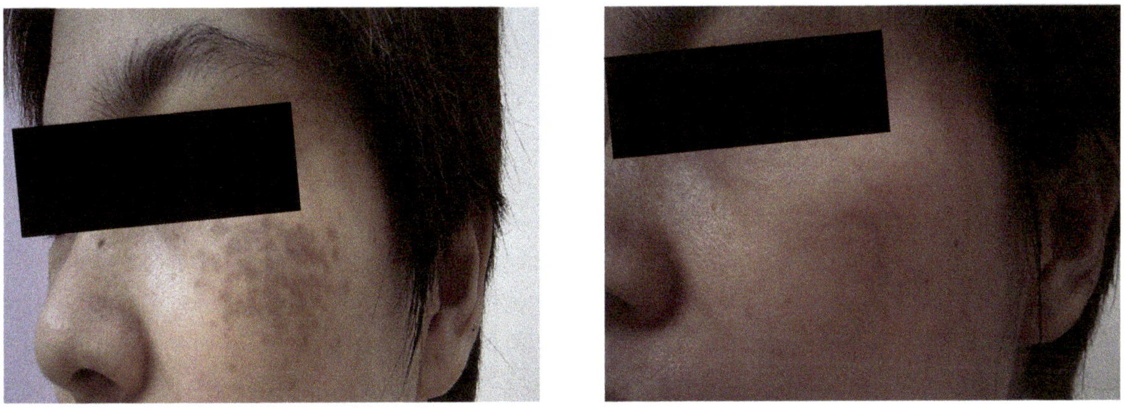

(a) (b)

Figure 5.12.

Case 12. Hori's nevus. (a) Before treatment. (b) After 9 treatments with the QS 1,064 nm Nd:YAG laser at 3–4 monthly intervals: 3 mm spot, 10 J/cm^2.

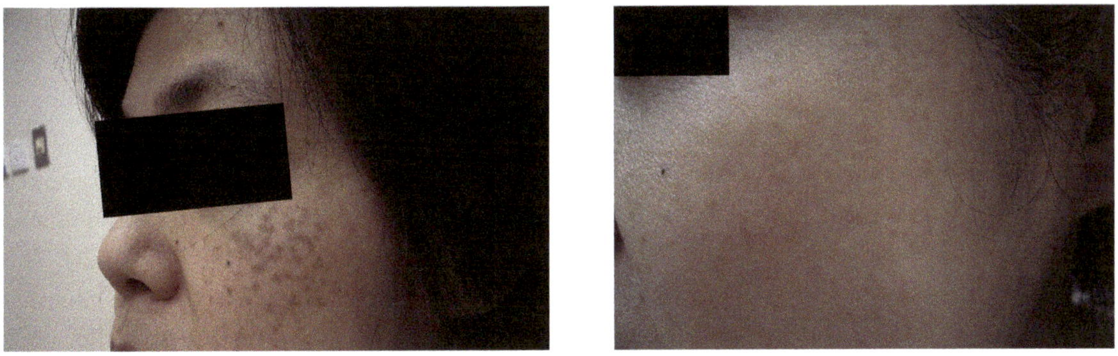

(a) (b)

Figure 5.13.

Case 13. Hori's nevus. (a) Before treatment. (b) After 10 treatments with the QS 1,064 nm Nd:YAG laser at 3–4 monthly intervals: 3 mm spot, 10 J/cm^2.

use of topical bleaching agents like hydroquinone and tretinoin to discharge epidermal melanin 4–6 weeks prior to Q-switched ruby laser was effective in Hori's nevus with a low rate of PIH and decreased the number of laser sessions.[3,86]

Other combination treatments include the use of the scanned CO_2 laser to remove the epidermis followed by the Q-switched ruby laser has been shown to be more effective than Q-switched ruby laser alone in the treatment of Hori's nevus.[87] Ee *et al.* showed that the combination of Q-switched 532 nm Nd:YAG laser (to remove epidermal hyperpigmentation) followed by the Q-switched 1064 nm Nd:YAG (532 nm, 4 mm spot, 1.2 J/cm^2; and 1064 nm, 4 mm spot, 6.5 J/cm^2) was more effective than Q-switched 1064 nm Nd:YAG laser alone for Hori's nevus.[88]

Congenital Melanocytic Nevus

Congenital melanocytic nevi are present in 1% of newborns.[89] The standard of care is surgical excision with histology, as there is an increased risk of melanoma developing in these lesions, with the reported lifetime risk ranging from 4.5–8.5% in patients with large congenital melanocytic nevi.[90,91] Prophylactic complete excision of large congenital melanocytic nevi is ideal but seldom achievable. Laser treatment of melanocytic nevi is controversial, as it is unclear whether repeated exposures to sub-lethal laser energy predispose cells to malignant change, but this is countered by the possibility that the decreased nevus load may decrease this risk. In some situations, the congenital melanocytic nevus may occur in functionally or cosmetically sensitive areas such as the face, perineum, hands, or feet, where surgical excision is not an option or may leave disfiguring scars.[92] Lasers have increasingly been used in such situations.

The Q-switched ruby,[93] the Q-switched alexandrite,[94] and the Q-switched 1064 nm Nd:YAG[95] lasers have been used to treat congenital melanocytic nevi with variable results. The Q-switched ruby and the Q-switched alexandrite lasers appeared to be more effective than the Q-switched 1064 nm Nd:YAG laser in lightening the nevi.[94,95] Although Q-switched lasers may lighten congenital nevi after multiple sessions, there is a high rate of repigmentation due to persistence of nevomelanocytes in the deeper reticular dermis.[93–95]

Congenital nevi consist of pigmented cells that are clustered in relatively large nests and it has been proposed that the poor results of the Q-switched lasers are due to failure to eradicate all the cells of the nest.[96] The long-pulse (ms) duration of the normal mode lasers produces more heat, which radiates to the surrounding cells and destroys complete nests of melanocytes rather than individual pigmented cells (Fig. 5.14). Impressive long-term reduction in pigmentation and hair growth in congenital nevi was achieved using the millisecond normal mode ruby laser. Long-term follow-up for at least eight years after laser treatment showed no evidence of malignant change.[97] The good cosmetic result was due to the presence of a subtle microscopic scar masking the underlying residual nevus cells. Combined normal mode ruby laser and Q-switched ruby laser have also been used to treat congenital melanocytic nevi, with good results after multiple sessions.[98,99] Ablation of the superficial pigment was performed initially in the Q-switched mode, which subsequently enhanced the penetration of the normal mode ruby laser.[98] Kono *et al.* used the normal mode ruby laser to first remove the epidermis, followed immediately by multiple passes with the Q-switched ruby laser. They found that the superficial intradermal type of congenital melanocytic nevus on histology had the best response.[99]

Resurfacing lasers like the erbium:YAG (Fig. 5.15) have been used to treat inoperable congenital melanocytic nevi, with good results.[100,101] Multiple treatments are needed at 4–9 monthly intervals.[100] As the deep dermal melanocytes are not ablated with the erbium:YAG laser, there is a tendency for incomplete clearance and recurrence, requiring treatments at regular intervals to maintain response. Combination CO_2 lasers and Q-switched pigment-specific lasers have also been used to treat congenital melanocytic nevi effectively.[102,103] The CO_2 laser removes the epidermis, which reduces the scattering of the beam, allowing the pigment-specific lasers to target the dermal melanocytes more effectively.

All these laser-treated patients require long-term follow-up with routine palpation of the treated areas to try to detect any subcutaneous changes. Any signs of recurrence or change should be carefully approached by considering a skin biopsy.[97]

Conclusion

Laser treatments in the Asian skin can be undertaken effectively and safely with proper patient selection and

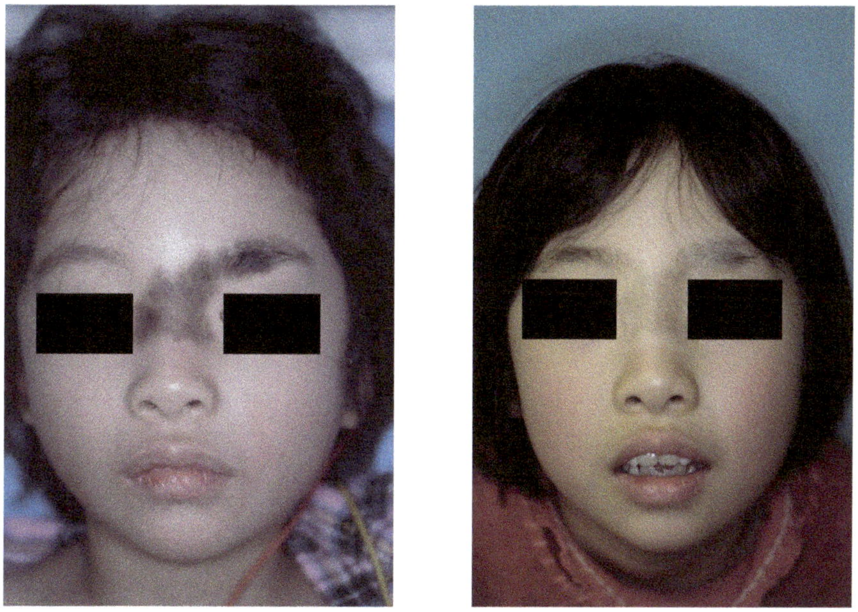

(a) (b)

Figure 5.14.

Case 14. Congenital melanocytic nevus. (a) Before treatment. (b) After 5 treatments with the long pulsed alexandrite laser, 20 J/cm^2 followed immediately by the QS alexandrite laser, 7 J/cm^2. (Courtesy of Taro Kono, MD, PhD, Tokyo, Japan.)

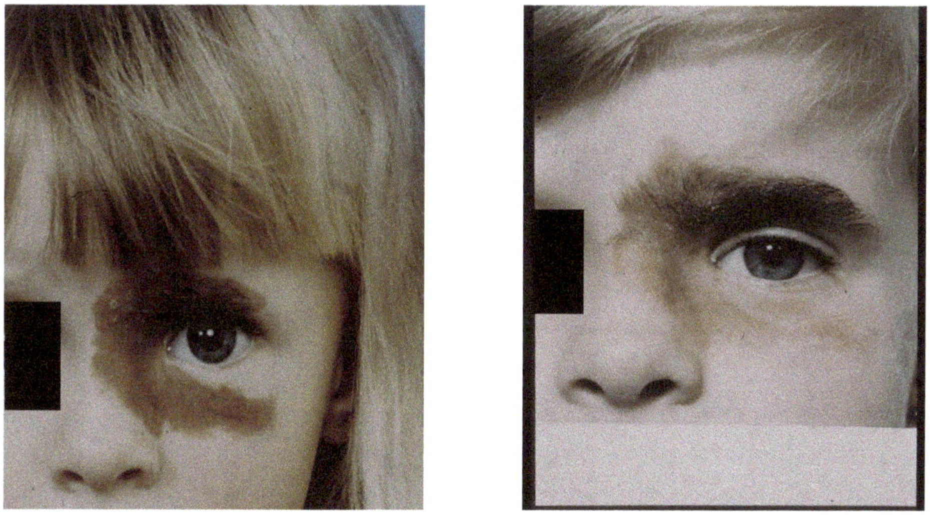

(a) (b)

Figure 5.15.

Case 15. Congenital melanocytic nevus. (a) Before treatment. (b) After 2 erbium:YAG resurfacing treatments to the inferior half of the lesion: 2940 nm, 5 mm spot, 300 ms, 400–450 mJ/cm^2 at 6–9 months apart. (Courtesy of Abdullah A, FRCP, Birmingham, UK.)

understanding of laser parameters, e.g. use of longer wavelength, longer pulse duration in the treatment of some pigmented lesions, more conservative fluences, and epidermal cooling to minimize damage to the epidermis. The use of pre- and postoperative bleaching skin care regimen is essential to the success of the procedure.

References

1. Alaluf S, Atkins D, Barrett K, *et al.* (2002) Ethnic variation in melanin content and composition in photoexposed and photoprotected human skin. *Pigment Cell Res* **15**: 112–118.
2. Goh SH. (1990) The treatment of visible signs of senescence: the Asian experience. *Br J Dermatol* **122** (Suppl. 35): 105–109.
3. Yoshimura K, Sato K, Aiba-Kojima E, *et al.* (2006) Repeated treatment protocols for melasma and acquired dermal melanocytosis. *Dermatol Surg* **32**: 365–371.
4. Espinal-Perez LE, Moncada B, Castanedo-Cazares JP. (2004) A double-blind randomized trial of 5% ascorbic acid vs 4% hydroquinone in melasma. *Int J Dermatol* **43**: 604–607.
5. Polla LL, Margolis RJ, Dover JS, *et al.* (1987) Melanosomes are a primary target of Q-switched ruby laser irradiation in guinea pig skin. *J Invest Dermatol* **89**: 281–286.
6. Anderson RR, Parrish JA. (1981) The optics of human skin. *J Invest Dermatol* **77**: 13–19.
7. Anderson RR, Parrish JA. (1983) Selective photothermolysis: precise microsurgery by selective absorption of pulsed radiation. *Science* **220**: 524–527.
8. Stratigos AJ, Dover JS, Arndt KA. (2000) Laser treatment of pigmented lesions-2000. How far have we gone? *Arch Dermatol* **136**: 915–921.
9. Taylor CR, Anderson RR. (1994) Ineffective treatment of refractory melasma and postinflammatory hyperpigmentation by Q-switched ruby laser. *J Dermatol Surg Oncol* **20**: 592–597.
10. Hruza GJ, Dover JS, Flotte TJ, *et al.* (1991) Q-switched ruby laser irradiation of normal human skin. Histologic and ultrastructural findings. *Arch Dermatol* **127**: 1799–1805.
11. Chung JH. (2003) Photoaging in Asians. *Photodermatol Photoimmunol Photomed* **19**: 109–121.
12. Goldberg DJ. (1993) Benign pigmented lesions of the skin. Treatment with the Q-switched ruby laser. *J Dermatol Surg Oncol* **19**: 376–379.
13. Wang CC, Sue YM, Yang CH, *et al.* (2006) A comparison of Q-switched alexandrite laser and intense pulsed light for the treatment of freckles and lentigines in Asian persons: a randomized, physician-blinded, split-face comparative trial. *J Am Acad Dermatol* **54**: 804–810.
14. Suh DH, Han KH, Chung JH. (2001) The use of Q-switched Nd:YAG laser in the treatment of superficial pigmented lesions in Koreans. *J Dermatol Treat* **12**: 91–96.
15. Sadighha A, Saatee S, Muhaghegh-Zahed G. (2008) Efficacy and adverse effects of Q-switched ruby laser on solar lentigines: a prospective study of 91 patients with Fitzpatrick skin type II, III and IV. *Dermatol Surg* **34**: 1465–1468.
16. Tse Y, Levine VJ, Mcclain SA, *et al.* (1994) The removal of cutaneous pigmented lesions with the Q-switched ruby laser and the Q-switched Neodymium: Yttrium-Aluminum-Garnet laser. *J Dermatol Surg Oncol* **20**: 795–800.
17. DePadova-Elder SM, Milgraum SS. (1994) Q-switched ruby laser treatment of labial lentigines in Peutz-Jeghers syndrome. *J Dermatol Surg Oncol* **20**: 830–832.
18. Gupta G, MacKay IR, Mackie RM. (1999) Q-switched ruby laser in the treatment of labial melanotic macules. *Lasers Surg Med* **25**: 219–222.
19. Papadavid E, Walker NPJ. (2001) Q-switched Alexandrite laser in the treatment of pigmented macules in Laugier-Hunziker syndrome. *J Eur Acad Dermatol Venereol* **15**: 468–469.
20. Xi Z, Hui Q, Zhong L. (2009) Q-switched Alexandrite laser treatment of oral labial lentigines in Chinese subjects with Peutz-Jeghers syndrome. *Dermatol Surg* **35**: 1084–1088.
21. Poon VK, Huang L, Burd A. (2005) Biostimulation of dermal fibroblast by 532 nm sublethal Q-switched Nd:YAG 532 nm laser: collagen remodeling and pigmentation. *J Photochem Photobiol B* **81**: 1–8.
22. Chan HHL. (2005) Effective and safe use of lasers, light sources and radiofrequency devices in the clinical management of Asian patients with selected dermatoses. *Lasers Surg Med* **37**: 179–185.
23. Chan HH, Fung WKK, Ying SY, *et al.* (2000) An in vivo trial comparing the use of different types of 532 nm Nd:YAG lasers in the treatment of facial lentigines in Oriental patients. *Dermatol Surg* **26**: 743–749.
24. Rashid T, Hussain I, Haider M, *et al.* (2002) Laser therapy of freckles and lentigines with quasi-continuous, frequency-doubled, Nd:YAG (532 nm) laser in Fitzpatrick skin type IV: a 24-month follow up. *J Cosmet Laser Ther* **4**: 81–85.

25. Rosenbach A, Lee SJ, Johr RH. (2002) Treatment of medium-brown solar lentigines using an alexandrite laser designed for hair reduction. *Arch Dermatol* **138**: 547–548.
26. Trafeli JP, Kwan JM, Meehan KJ, *et al.* (2007) Use of a long-pulse alexandrite laser in the treatment of superficial pigmented lesions. *Dermatol Surg* **33**: 1477–1482.
27. Kono T, Manstein D, Chan HH, *et al.* (2006) Q-switched ruby versus long-pulsed dye laser delivered with compression for treatment of facial lentigines in Asians. *Lasers Surg Med* **38**: 94–97.
28. Grossman MC, Anderson RR, Farinelli W, *et al.* (1995) Treatment of café au lait macules with lasers. A clinicopathologic correlation. *Arch Dermatol* **131**: 1416–1420.
29. Kagami S, Asahina A, Watanabe R, *et al.* (2007) Treatment of 153 Japanese patients with Q-switched alexandrite laser. *Lasers Med Sci* **22**: 159–163.
30. Alster TS. (1995) Complete elimination of large café-au-lait birthmarks by 510-nm pulsed dye laser. *Plast Reconstr Surg* **96**: 1660–1664.
31. Somyos K, Boonchu K, Somsak K, *et al.* (1996) Copper vapour laser treatment of café-au-lait macules. *Br J Dermatol* **135**: 964–968.
32. Alora MB, Arndt KA. (2001) Treatment of a café-au-lai macule with the erbium: YAG laser. *J Am Acad Dermatol* **45**: 566–568.
33. Kim JS, Kim MJ, Cho SB. (2009) Treatment of segmental café-au-lait macules using 1064-nm Q-switched Nd:YAG laser with low pulse energy. *Clin Exp Dermatol* **34**: e223–e224.
34. Shimbashi T, Kamide R, Hashimoto T. (1997) Long-term follow-up in treatment of solar lentigo and café-au-lait macules with Q-switched ruby laser. *Aesthetic Plast Surg* **21**: 445–448.
35. Grevelink JM, Gonzalez S, Bonoan R, *et al.* (1997) Treatment of nevus spilus with the Q-switched ruby laser. *Dermatol Surg* **23**: 365–370.
36. Taylor CR, Anderson RR. (1993) Treatment of benign pigmented epidermal lesions by Q-switched ruby laser. *Int J Dermatol* **32**: 908–912.
37. Moreno-Arias GA, Bulla F, Vilata-Corell JJ, *et al.* (2001) Treatment of widespread segmental nevus spilus by Q-switched alexandrite laser (755 nm, 100 nsec). *Dermatol Surg* **27**: 841–843.
38. Danarti R, König A, Salhi A, *et al.* (2004) Becker's nevus syndrome revisited. *J Am Acad Dermatol* **51**: 965–969.
39. Trelles MA, Allones I, Moreno-Arias GA, *et al.* (2005) Becker's naevus: a comparative study between erbium:YAG and Q-switched neodymium:YAG; clinical and histopathological findings. *Br J Dermatol* **152**: 308–313.
40. Nanni CA, Alster TS. (1998) Treatment of a Becker's nevus using a 694-nm long-pulsed ruby laser. *Dermatol Surg* **24**: 1032–1034.
41. Choi JE, Kim JW, Seo SH, *et al.* (2009) Treatment of Becker's nevi with a long-pulse alexandrite laser. *Dermatol Surg* **35**: 1105–1108.
42. Glaich AS, Goldberg LH, Dai T, *et al.* (2007) Fractional resurfacing: a new therapeutic modality for Becker's nevus. *Arch Dermatol* **143**: 1488–1490.
43. Gupta AK, Gover MD, Nouri K, *et al.* (2006) The treatment of melasma: a review of clinical trials. *J Am Acad Dermatol* **55**: 1048–1065.
44. Sanchez NP, Pathak MA, Sato S, *et al.* (1981) Melasma: a clinical, light microscopic, ultrastructural, and immunofluorescence study. *J Am Acad Dermatol* **4**: 698–710.
45. Kang WH, Yoon KH, Lee ES, *et al.* (2002) Melasma: histopathological characteristics in 56 Korean patients. *Br J Dermatol* **146**: 228–237.
46. Salem A, Gamil H, Ramadan A, *et al.* (2009) Melasma: treatment evaluation. *J Cosmet Laser Ther* **11**: 146–150.
47. Rendon M, Berneburg M, Arellano I, *et al.* (2006) Treatment of melasma. *J Am Acad Dermatol* **54**: S272–S281.
48. Rusciani A, Motta A, Rusciani L, *et al.* (2005) Q-switched alexandrite laser-assisted treatment of melasma: 2-year follow-up monitoring. *J Drugs Dermatol* **4**: 770–774.
49. Polnikorn N. (2008) Treatment of refractory dermal melasma with the Medite C6 Q-switched Nd:YAG laser: two case reports. *J Cosmet Laser Ther* **10**: 167–173.
50. Cho SB, Kim JS, Kim MJ. (2009) Melasma treatment in Korean women using a 1064-nm Q-switched Nd:YAG laser with low pulse energy. *Clin Exp Dermatol* **34**: e847–850.
51. Kim MJ, Kim JS, Cho SB. (2009) Punctuate leucoderma after melasma treatment using 1064-nm Q-switched Nd:YAG laser with low pulse energy. *J Eur Acad Dermatol Venereol* **23**: 960–962.
52. Manaloto RMP, Alster T. (1999) Erbium:YAG laser resurfacing for refractory melasma. *Dermatol Surg* **25**: 121–123.
53. Wanitphakdeedecha R, Manuskiatti W, Siriphukpong S, *et al.* (2009) Treatment of melasma using variable square pulse Er:YAG laser resurfacing. *Dermatol Surg* **35**: 475–482.
54. Nouri K, Bowes L, Chartier T, *et al.* (1999) Combination treatment of melasma with pulsed CO_2 laser followed by

Q-switched alexandrite laser: a pilot study. *Dermatol Surg* **25**: 494–497.

55. Angsuwarangsee S, Polnikorn N. (2003) Combined ultrapulse CO_2 laser and Q-switched alexandrite laser compared with Q-switched alexandrite laser alone for refractory melasma: split-face design. *Dermatol Surg* **29**: 59–64.
56. Tannous ZS, Astner S. (2005) Utilizing fractional resurfacing in the treatment of therapy-resistant melasma. *J Cosmet Laser Ther* **7**: 39–43.
57. Rokhsar CK, Fitzpatrick RE. (2005) The treatment of melasma with fractional photothermolysis: a pilot study. *Dermatol Surg* **31**: 1645–1650.
58. Naito SK. (2007) Fractional photothermolysis treatment for resistant melasma in Chinese females. *J Cosmet Laser Ther* **9**: 161–163.
59. Lee HS, Won CH, Lee DH, *et al.* (2009) Treatment of melasma in Asian skin using a fractional 1,550-nm laser: an open clinical study. *Dermatol Surg* **35**: 1499–1504.
60. Hantash BM, Bedi VP, Sudireddy V, *et al.* (2006) Laser-induced transepidermal elimination of dermal content by fractional photothermolysis. *J Biomed Opt* **11**: 041115.
61. Goldberg DJ, Berlin AL, Phelps R. (2008) Histologic and ultrastructural analysis of melasma after fractional resurfacing. *Lasers Surg Med* **40**: 134–138.
62. Teekhasaenee C, Ritch R, Rutnin U, *et al.* (1990) Glaucoma in oculodermal melanocytosis. *Ophthalmology* **97**: 562–570.
63. Patel BC, Egan CA, Lucius RW, *et al.* (1998) Cutaneous malignant melanoma and oculodermal melanocytosis (nevus of Ota): report of a case and review of the literature. *J Am Acad Dermatol* **38**: 862–865.
64. Wang HW, Liu YH, Zhang GK, *et al.* (2007) Analysis of 602 Chinese cases of nevus of Ota and the treatment results treated by Q-switched alexandrite laser. *Dermatol Surg* **33**: 455–460.
65. Mataix J, Lopez N, Haro R, *et al.* (2007) Late-onset Ito's nevus: an uncommon acquired dermal melanocytosis. *J Cutan Pathol* **34**: 640–643.
66. Goldberg DJ, Nychay SG. (1992) Q-switched ruby laser treatment of nevus of Ota. *J Dermatol Surg Oncol* **18**: 817–821.
67. Geronemus RG. (1992) Q-switched ruby laser therapy of nevus of Ota. *Arch Dermatol* **128**: 1618–1622.
68. Moreno-Arias GA, Camps-Fresneda A. (2001) Treatment of nevus of Ota with the Q-switched alexandrite laser. *Lasers Surg Med* **28**: 451–455.
69. Zhong L, Lihua F, Sheng J, *et al.* (2003) Treatment of 522 patients with nevus of Ota with Q-switched alexandrite laser. *Chin Med J* **116**: 226–230.
70. Apfelberg DB. (1995) Argon and Q-switched Yttrium-Aluminium-Garnet laser treatment of nevus of Ota. *Ann Plast Surg* **35**: 150–153.
71. Chan HH, Ying SY, Ho WS, *et al.* (2000) An in vivo trial comparing the clinical efficacy and complications of Q-switched 755 nm alexandrite and Q-switched 1064 nm Nd:YAG lasers in the treatment of nevus of Ota. *Dermatol Surg* **26**: 919–922.
72. Ueda S, Isoda M, Imayama S. (2000) Response of naevus of Ota to Q-switched ruby laser treatment according to lesion colour. *Br J Dermatol* **142**: 77–83.
73. Kono T, Chan HH, Ercöcen AR, *et al.* (2003) Use of Q-switched ruby laser in the treatment of nevus of Ota in different age groups. *Lasers Surg Med* **32**: 391–395.
74. Chan HH, Leung RSC, Ying SY, *et al.* (2000) Recurrence of nevus of Ota after successful treatment with Q-switched lasers. *Arch Dermatol* **136**: 1175–1176.
75. Chan HH, Leung RSC, Ying SY, *et al.* (2000) A retrospective analysis of complications in the treatment of nevus of Ota with the Q-switched alexandrite and Q-switched Nd:YAG lasers. *Dermatol Surg* **26**: 1000–1006.
76. Kouba DJ, Fincher EF, Moy RL. (2008) Nevus of Ota successfully treated by fractional photothermolysis using a fractionated 1440-nm Nd:YAG laser. *Arch Dermatol* **144**: 156–158.
77. Hori Y, Kawashima M, Oohara K, *et al.* (1984) Acquired, bilateral nevus of Ota-like macules. *J Am Acad Dermatol* **10**: 961–964.
78. Ee HL, Wong HC, Goh CL, *et al.* (2006) Characteristics of Hori naevus: a prospective analysis. *Br J Dermatol* **154**: 50–53.
79. Park JM, Tsao H, Tsao S. (2009) Acquired bilateral nevus of Ota-like macules (Hori nevus): etiologic and therapeutic considerations. *J Am Acad Dermatol* **61**: 88–93.
80. Lee B, Kim YC, Kang WH, *et al.* (2004) Comparison of characteristics of acquired bilateral nevus of Ota-like macules and nevus of Ota according to therapeutic outcome. *J Korean Med Sci* **19**: 554–559.
81. Kunachak S, Leelaudomlipi P, Sirikulchayanonta V. (1999) Q-switched ruby laser therapy of acquired bilateral nevus of Ota-like macules. *Dermatol Surg* **25**: 938–941.
82. Lam AYM, Wong DSY, Lam LK, *et al.* (2001) A retrospective study on the efficacy and complications of Q-switched alexandrite laser in the treatment of acquired bilateral nevus of Ota-like macules. *Dermatol Surg* **27**: 937–942.

83. Kunachak S, Leelaudomlipi P. (2000) Q-switched Nd:YAG laser treatment for acquired bilateral nevus of Ota-like maculae: a long-term follow-up. *Lasers Surg Med* **26**: 376–379.
84. Polnikorn N, Tanrattanakorn S, Goldberg DJ. (2000) Treatment of Hori's nevus with the Q-switched Nd:YAG laser. *Dermatol Surg* **26**: 477–480.
85. Suh DH, Han KH, Chung JH. (2001) Clinical use of the Q-switched Nd:YAG laser for the treatment of acquired bilateral nevus of Ota-like macules (ABNOMs) in Koreans. *J Dermatol Treat* **12**: 163–166.
86. Momosawa A, Yoshimura K, Uchida G, *et al.* (2003) Combined therapy using Q-switched ruby laser and bleaching treatment with tretinoin and hydroquinone for acquired dermal melanocytosis. *Dermatol Surg* **29**: 1001–1007.
87. Manuskiatti W, Sivayathorn A, Leelaudomlipi P, *et al.* (2003) Treatment of acquired bilateral nevus of Ota-like macules (Hori's nevus) using a combination of scanned carbon dioxide laser followed by Q-switched ruby laser. *J Am Acad Dermatol* **48**: 584–591.
88. Ee HL, Goh CL, Khoo L, *et al.* (2006) Treatment of acquired bilateral nevus of Ota-like macules (Hori's nevus) with a combination of the 532 nm Q-switched Nd:YAG laser followed by the 1,064 nm Q-switched Nd:YAG is more effective: prospective study. *Dermatol Surg* **32**: 34–40.
89. Walton RG, Jacobs AH, Cox AJ. (1976) Pigmented lesions in newborn infants. *Br J Dermatol* **95**: 389–396.
90. Rhodes AR, Sober AJ, Day CL, *et al.* (1982) The malignant potential of small congenital nevocellular nevi. An estimate of association based on a histologic study of 234 primary cutaneous melanomas. *J Am Acad Dermatol* **6**: 230–241.
91. Bittencourt FV, Marghoob AA, Kopf AW, *et al.* (2000) Large congenital melanocytic nevi and the risk for development of malignant melanoma and neurocutaneous melanocytosis. *Pediatrics* **106**: 736–741.
92. Watt AJ, Kotsis SV, Chung KC. (2004) Risk of melanoma arising in large congenital melanocytic nevi: a systematic review. *Plast Reconstr Surg* **113**: 1968–1974.
93. Waldorf HA, Kauvar ANB, Geronemus RG. (1996) Treatment of small and medium congenital nevi with the Q-switched ruby laser. *Arch Dermatol* **132**: 301–304.
94. Rosenbach A, Williams CM, Alster TS. (1997) Comparison of the Q-switched alexandrite (755 nm) and Q-switched Nd:YAG (1064 nm) lasers in the treatment of benign melanocytic nevi. *Dermatol Surg* **23**: 239–245.
95. Grevelink JM, van Leeuwen RL, Anderson RR, *et al.* (1997) Clinical and histological responses of congenital melanocytic nevi after single treatment with Q-switched lasers. *Arch Dermatol* **133**: 349–353.
96. Ueda S, Imayama S. (1997) Normal-mode ruby laser for treating congenital nevi. *Arch Dermatol* **133**: 355–359.
97. Imayama S, Ueda S. (1999) Long-and short-term histological observations of congenital nevi treated with thenormal-mode ruby laser. *Arch Dermatol* **135**: 1211–1218.
98. Noordzij MJ, van den Broecke DG, Alting MC, *et al.* (2004) Ruby laser treatment of congenital melanocytic nevi: a review of the literature and report of our own experience. *Plast Reconstr Surg* **114**: 660–667.
99. Kono T, Ercöcen AR, Nozaki M. (2005) Treatment of congenital melanocytic nevi using the combined (normal-mode plus Q-switched) ruby laser in Asians clinical response in relation to histological type. *Ann Plast Surg* **54**: 494–501.
100. Rajpar SF, Abdullah A, Lanigan SW. (2006) Er:YAG laser resurfacing for inoperable medium-sized facial congenital mel-anocytic naevi in children. *Clin Exp Dermatol* **32**: 159–161.
101. Ostertag JU, Quaedvlieg PJF, Kerckhoffs FEMJ, *et al.* (2006) Congenital naevi treated with erbium:YAG laser (Derma K) resurfacing in neonates: clinical results and review of the literature. *Br J Dermatol* **154**: 889–895.
102. Chong SJ, Jeong E, Park HJ, *et al.* (2005) Treatment of congenital nevomelanocytic nevi with the CO_2 and Q-switched alexandrite lasers. *Dermatol Surg* **31**: 518–521.
103. Dave R, Mahaffey PJ. (2004) Combined early treatment of congenital melanocytic naevus with carbon dioxide and NdYag lasers. *Br J Plast Surg* **57**: 720–724.

Chapter 6

Laser Treatment of Tattoos

Eileen Tan*

Introduction

Tattoos can be dated back to prehistory. There is a paucity of demographic data on tattoos in the Asian population although there are various studies from the West.[1–4] Some of the reasons for the increasing popularity of tattooing in the United States include peer pressure and improved self image.[1,2] Reasons for tattoo removal include dissociation from the past and a shift in the patient's identity. In our experience, tattooing is becoming more common among the young in Singapore as a result of increasing urbanization and Westernization. The focus of this chapter will cover the various types of tattoos and the laser treatment options for removing tattoos with emphasis on Asian skin types.

Non-laser tattoo removal methods include dermabrasion,[5] cryosurgery,[6] and excision.[7] Tattoo removal by laser was performed with continuous wave lasers initially,[8,9] and later improved with Q-switched lasers in the 1990s. Presently, laser tattoo removal usually refers to the noninvasive removal of tattoo pigments using Q-switched lasers.[10–12]

Categories of Tattoos[13] (Table 6.1)

Professional Tattoos

Professional tattoos are applied by registered artists using a tattoo machine or a tattoo gun. These tattoos are composed of one or several colors of organometallic dyes (Fig. 6.1). Large amounts of ink are uniformly injected into the dermis to create a sharp and clear image. Professional tattoos often contain multiple pigments that require more treatments to clear.

Amateur Tattoos

Amateur tattoos are made by individuals or their friends jabbing ink, charcoal, or ashes under the skin with a pin. An amateur tattoo usually appears gray or blue-black in color (Fig. 6.2). The resultant tattoo is not as sharp or well defined as a professional tattoo. Amateur tattoos usually require fewer laser treatments to remove because they usually consist of a single pigment.

Cosmetic Tattoos

Cosmetic tattoos are commonly performed in beauty parlors. In general, black, brown, and red inks are employed as "permanent make-up" to create lipliner, eyeliner, and eyebrows, etc. (Fig. 6.3).

Traumatic Tattoos

Traumatic tattoos occur during mechanical penetration of the skin by foreign body particles such as carbon-containing material, dirt, or other materials (Fig. 6.4). The ease of removal depends on the depth of the penetration of the substance.

*Consultant Dermatologist, Eileen Tan Skin, Laser and Hair Transplant Clinic, Mount Elizabeth Medical Centre, Singapore.

Table 6.1.

Tattoo Categorization

Tattoo Types	Pigment Type	Ink Concentration	Pigment Depth
Professional	Organometallic dyes	Dense	Deep
Amateur	India ink (carbon)	Sparse	Variable
Cosmetic	Iron or titanium oxide	Sparse	Superficial
Traumatic	Carbon, metals, dirt	Variable	Variable
Medicinal	India ink (carbon)	Sparse	Superficial

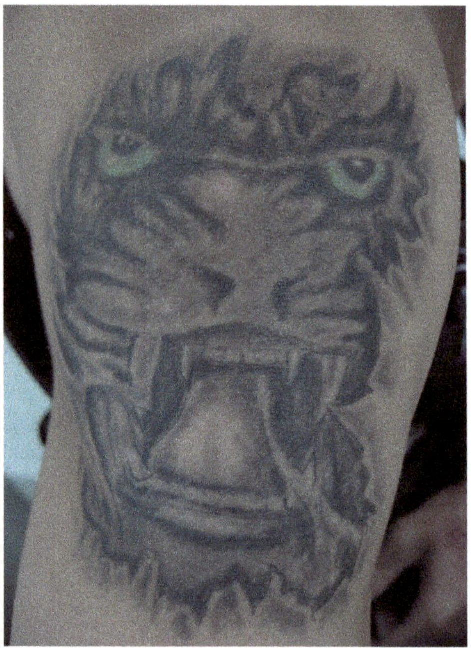

Figure 6.1.

An example of a multicolored professional tattoo.

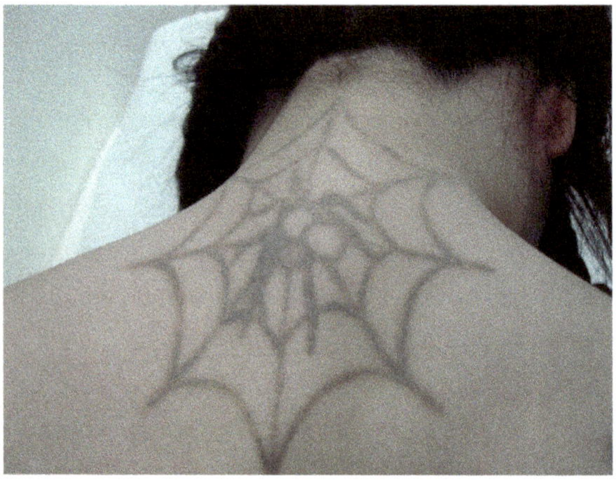

Figure 6.2.

An example of a black amateur tattoo.

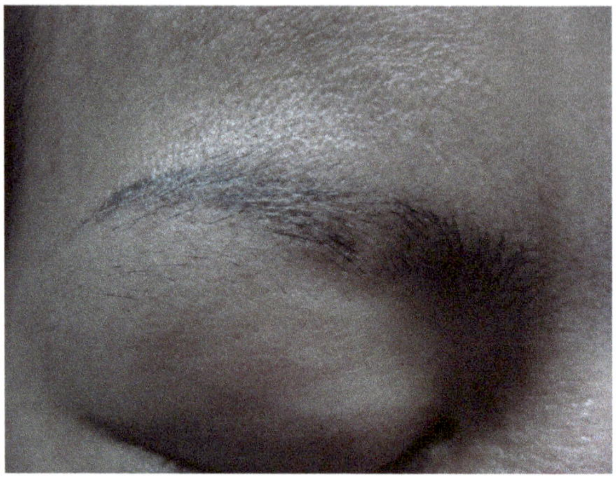

Figure 6.3.

Partially removed black cosmetic eyebrow tattoo.

Medicinal Tattoos

These are iatrogenic tattoos inserted as part of research identification or therapeutic indications. They are generally superficial blue-black tattoos measuring 1–3 mm in diameter.[14]

Pathogenesis of Tattoo Laser Removal

In tattoo removal, the target for the laser light consists of small particles of tattoo ink that are found either within macrophages or scattered extracellularly throughout the dermis. These tattoo inks are, in general, too large to be removed from the skin. Laser treatment causes tattoo pigment particles to heat up and fragment into smaller pieces. These smaller pieces are then removed by normal body processes.[14,15]

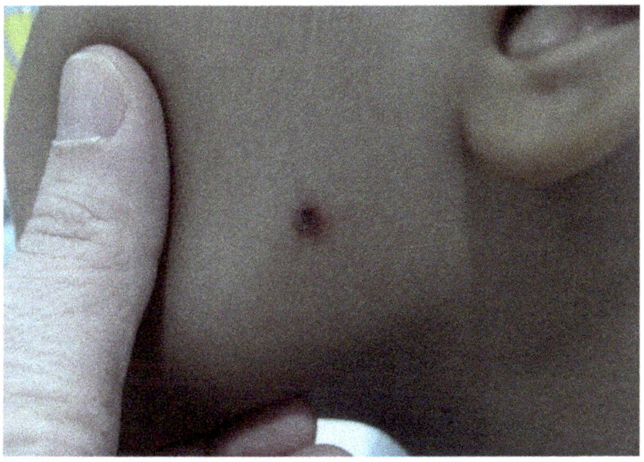

Figure 6.4.

A 6-year-old boy with a traumatic tattoo due to pencil lead injury.

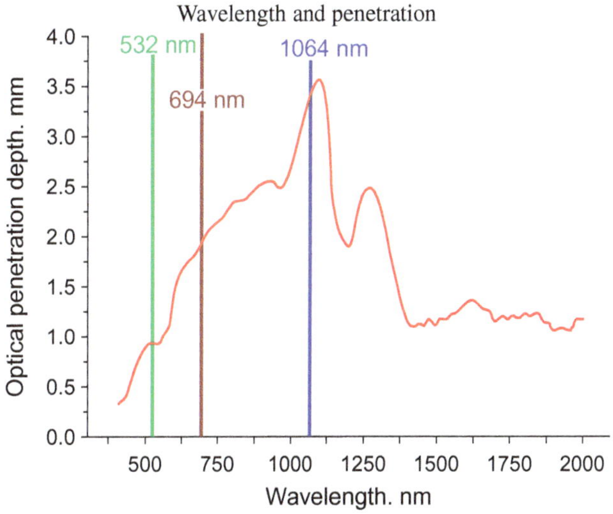

Figure 6.5.

Optimal penetration depth (mm) for various laser systems (wavelength in nanometers).

Several tattoo-specific lasers are available (Table 6.2). Treatment of tattoos with lasers depends on the type of tattoo and its pigment content, as different lasers target different colored pigments (Fig. 6.5). Based on the principle of selective photothermolysis, the optimal wavelength achieves selective absorption for each particular ink color while minimizing scarring and damage to the surrounding skin.[16,17]

Q-switched Ruby Laser (694 nm)

This laser creates a red light that is highly absorbed by green and dark tattoo pigments. Red and yellow tattoo pigments do not respond to Q-switched ruby laser.[18–22] Clinical research has shown that short pulse durations of 25 nanoseconds (ns) and higher fluences of 8–10 J/cm^2 clear tattoos fairly rapidly. Kilmer and Anderson reported excellent clearance of black and green tattoos with treatment fluences of 6–8 J/cm^2 with a 40–80 ns pulse width.[22] Amateur tattoos usually require 4–6 treatment sessions and professional tattoos are usually cleared within 6–10 sessions. Professional and deeply placed tattoos may be more

Table 6.2.

Laser Treatment Options for Various Tattoo Inks

		Response			
Laser Type	**Parameters**	**Black Ink**	**Green Ink**	**Red Ink**	**Flesh-toned Ink**
QS Ruby	694 nm 25–50 ns	Excellent	Good	Poor	Usually blackens
QS Alexandrite	755 nm 50–100 ns	Excellent	Excellent	Poor	Usually blackens
QS Nd:YAG	1064 nm 10 ns	Excellent	Fair	Poor	Usually blackens
Frequency-doubled Nd:YAG	532 nm 10–40 ns	Poor	Poor	Excellent	Usually blackens

Adapted from Alster TS, Lewis AB. (1996) Dermatologic laser surgery: A review. *Dermatol Surg* **22**, 797–805.

difficult to eradicate. Acceptable clearing varies greatly from patient to patient as some individuals are more accepting of "shadowing," i.e. vague residual tattoo pigments.

As the Q-switched ruby laser is more highly absorbed by melanin, it often produces undesirable side effects such as pigmentary changes in patients with darker skin types. Scarring and textural changes occur more rarely.

Q-switched Alexandrite Laser (755 nm)

The alexandrite laser is highly absorbed by green and dark tattoo pigments. This laser is best at removing green tattoos but it is less effective than either the Q-switched ruby laser or Q-switched Nd:YAG laser at removing dark blue or black tattoos.[23–26] It is not effective for red tattoo inks. The alexandrite laser has a lower incidence of unwanted pigmentary changes because its wavelength is less absorbed by melanin.

Q-switched Nd:YAG Laser (532 nm and 1064 nm)

The Q-switched 1064 nm Nd:YAG laser is effective for the removal of black tattoos, with energies ranging from 5–10 J/cm^2 and 3 mm spot size. In comparison with the Q-switched ruby laser, the Q-switched Nd:YAG laser is more effective at treating black and dark tattoos because of its deeper penetration into the skin (Fig. 6.6). Several clinical studies have demonstrated that the Q-switched 1064 nm Nd:YAG laser is effective in removing Q-switched ruby laser resistant tattoos with a 2.5 mm spot size and fluences of 6–12 J/cm^2.[27–32] The frequency-doubled Q-switched Nd:YAG laser (532 nm) creates a green light that is highly absorbed by red targets. Hence it is effective in the treatment of red or orange color tattoos.

The Q-switched Nd:YAG laser offers an advantage for treating dark-skinned individuals. Effective tattoo removal with minimal pigmentary risks were demonstrated in clinical studies carried out by Grevelink *et al.*[12] and Jones *et al.*[28]

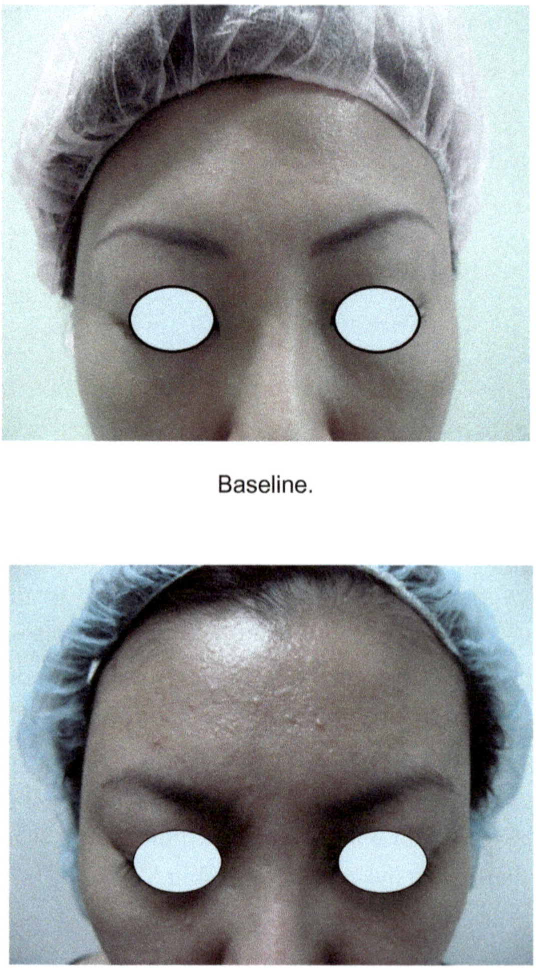

Baseline.

After 1 session of QS Nd:YAG laser using a 4 mm spot size and fluence of 4.2 J/cm^2, showing lightening of the tattoo.

Figure 6.6.

Eyebrow black tattoo treated with QS Nd:YAG laser (1064 nm).

Preoperative Patient Evaluation

There are increasing requests for tattoo removal from patients of all walks of life. In order to achieve treatment success, it is important to ascertain the patient's expectations and the appropriate laser treatment to achieve the desired clinical outcome.

Important points in history-taking and physical examination include the following:

1. *Type of tattoo*
   Typically, professional and multicolored tattoos are more difficult to remove because the tattoo ink is placed deeper and multiple colors are often employed. Several laser treatments are usually necessary.
   Some of the brown, rust-colored inks found in many cosmetic and professional tattoos are known to contain iron or titanium oxide pigment. These pigments can darken when undergoing Q-switched laser irradiation.
   Kirby *et al.* proposed a new tattoo scoring in 2009 to enable physicians to assess the feasibility of laser tattoo removal.[33] This scale can be used by the physician to assess the approximate number of treatments required. The Kirby-Desai Scale assigns numerical values to six parameters: skin type, location, color, amount of ink, scarring or tissue change, and layering. Parameter scores are then added to yield a combined score that will show the estimated number of treatments needed for successful tattoo removal.[33]
2. *Any contraindications to laser tattoo removal*
   Past history of poor wound healing, scarring, granulomatous, or allergic reactions should be carefully assessed. Individuals with darker skin phototypes run a higher risk of dyspigmentation, especially post-inflammatory hyperpigmentation. Additional laser treatments may be necessary.[34,35]

Treatment Procedure

Once suitability for tattoo laser removal has been established, the patient will need to understand appropriate pre- and postoperative instructions and give an informed consent. It is advisable to take photographs before starting treatment and periodically after a few laser sessions to assess the progress.

Most patients will require some form of local anesthesia. A commonly used topical anesthetic cream is EMLA®, which is a mixture containing lidocaine 2.5% and prilocaine 2.5%. Application of an anesthetic cream under occlusion for 45–90 minutes prior to the laser treatment session is a common practice. If complete anesthesia is desired, it can be administered locally by injections of 1–2% lidocaine with epinephrine.

All tattoo pigments have specific light absorption spectra. The physician should have a good understanding of the different laser devices as each laser system targets tattoo pigments selectively. Certain tattoo pigments, such as yellows, greens, and flesh-tone inks are more challenging to treat than the darker blacks and blues, because these pigments have absorption spectra that fall outside of the emission spectra available in the respective lasers.

Protective eyewear should be worn at all times during treatment. The treatment consists of placing a handpiece against the surface of the skin and activating the laser light. As many patients describe it, each pulse feels like a rubber band snapping against the skin. Immediately after the laser impact, a gray white appearance and pin-point bleeding of the treated sites are seen (clinical endpoint) (Fig. 6.7).

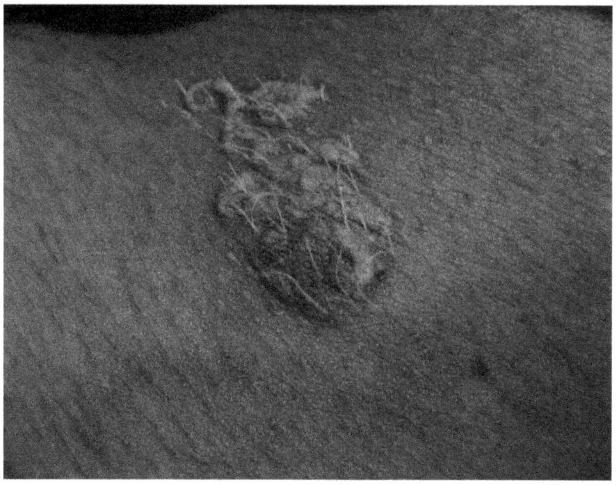

Figure 6.7.

Gray white appearance immediately after laser tattoo removal.

An ice pack is applied immediately to soothe the treated area. Edema and erythema usually resolve within 24–48 hours. Subsequently, crusting and sometimes blisters appear over the entire tattoo, which sloughs off and heals at approximately 7–14 days post treatment. Postoperative wound care consists of a topically applied antibiotic ointment and a non-occlusive dressing until healing occurs. Fading of the tattoo will be noted over the next 8–10 weeks, and subsequent treatment energy levels can be tailored depending on the clinical response observed.

With multiple treatments, tattoo lightening often occurs with little or no textural change. In general, laser treatments are delivered every 3–4 months to allow adequate wound healing and to faciliate clearance of tattoo fragments and cellular debris by the body's immune system.

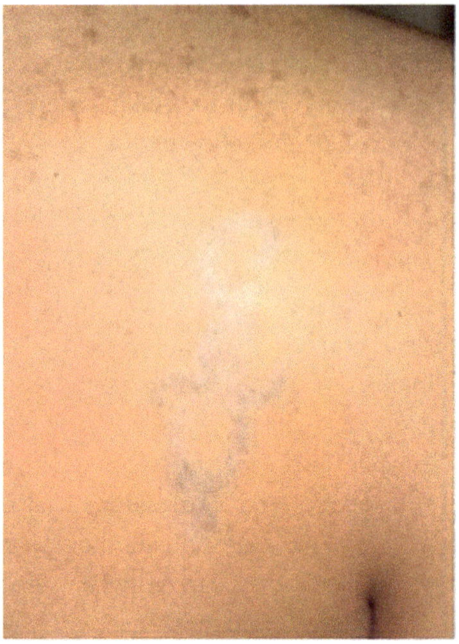

Figure 6.8.

Hypopigmentation that occurred after QS Nd:YAG laser treatment.

Side Effects and Complications

Alterations in Pigmentation

Dyspigmentation is a well-documented risk after laser treatment (Fig. 6.8). Studies have shown that people with darker Fitzpatrick skin types are more likely to be affected by post-inflammatory hyperpigmentation.[34–36] Thus, caution in individuals with darker skin (Fitzpatrick skin types IV–VI) should be exercised, using more conservative parameters regardless of the wavelength used. The underlying rationale is probably due to competitive absorption of the laser light by the higher melanin content found in the epidermis of ethnic skin.

About half of the patients treated with Q-switched lasers for tattoo removal will show some transient changes in the normal skin pigmentation. These changes usually resolve within 3–6 months but may rarely be permanent.[37] In general, post-inflammatory hyperpigmentation is easier to treat. It usually improves with broad spectrum sunscreens and topical bleaching creams such as 4% hydroquinone or Kligman's formulated products. It is advisable to wait until the post-inflammatory hyperpigmentation resolves before resuming laser treatments.

Hypopigmentation is more difficult to treat. Multiple sessions of localized narrow band ultraviolet light (UVB), excimer, or fractionated nonablative (1550 nm) laser may promote some degree of repigmentation.

Textural Changes and Scarring

Asian skin may be prone to develop hypertrophic or keloid scars post injury.[36,37] Hence, Asian patients and those with a past history of hypertrophic or keloidal scars must be warned of the increased risk of scarring. Scarring may be a sequel of secondary infection or if severe blistering and crusting of the tattoo site occurred post treatment. If an individual is prone to pigmentary or textural changes or if blistering has occurred, longer treatment intervals and lower fluences are recommended.

Darkening of Tattoo Pigments

Paradoxical darkening of flesh-tone, red, and white tattoo inks have been reported with Q-switched lasers (Fig. 6.9).

Darkening or blackening of the tattoo pigment is believed to result from the reduction of ferric oxide (rust color) to ferrous oxide (black color).[18,37,38] The underlying change is most likely due to an oxidation-reduction or the ignition of ferric oxide above 1400 degrees Celsius. Hence, extreme caution should be taken when considering laser treatment of cosmetic tattoos, especially those with red or flesh tones. The darkening effect may prove more difficult to remove and is certainly more visible than the original color tone. If the darkened area does not clear spontaneously, either repeated laser treatments or excision of the lesion may be necessary. The newly darkened tattoo can be treated as if it were black pigment about eight weeks from the initial laser session.

Test sites are recommended in high-risk individuals. It is suggested to retreat the darkened area immediately and wait several weeks to assess the clinical response. If it has lightened significantly, further treatment can be considered.

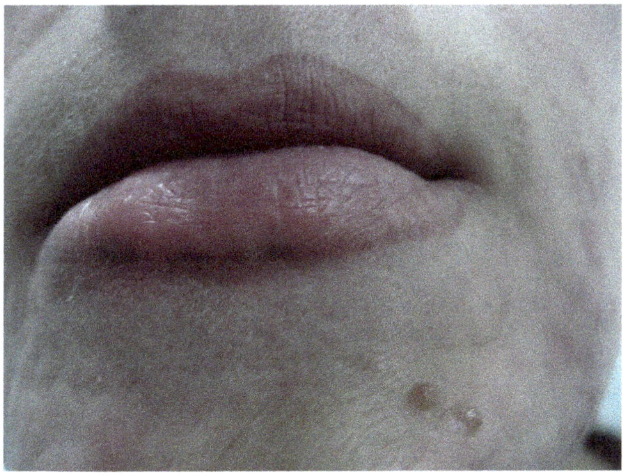

Figure 6.9.

Paradoxical darkening of a lip cosmetic tattoo after laser treatment.

Allergic Reactions and Tattoo Granuloma

Local allergic and granulomatous reactions have occurred in patients with multicolored tattoos.[39–44] These tattoos include yellow (cadmium), red (mercury), blue (cobalt), and green (cadmium) inks. The localized skin reaction, which consists of erythema, pruritus, inflammatory nodules, and granulomas, are confined to the site of the red/yellow ink. Treatment of tattoo granulomas consists of sunlight avoidance, use of sunscreen, intralesional steroid injections, and possibly surgical or CO_2 laser removal.

In rare instances, systemic allergic reactions can occur. Patients with prior allergic reactions are at a higher risk for a local or systemic reaction from laser-induced release of pigment antigens. Emergency anaphylactic precautions and premedication with antihistamines or systemic corticosteroids should be taken in these high-risk patients.

Conclusion

Q-switched lasers are highly effective in treating dark blue, black, green, and red tattoos. In the future, picosecond lasers will be developed so that other exotic colors may be treated with fewer sessions and without significant scarring or dyspigmentation.

References

1. Armstrong ML, Stuppy DJ, Gabriel DC, *et al.* (1996) Motivation for tattoo removal. *Arch Dermatol* **132**: 412–416.
2. Armstrong ML, Roberts AE, Koch JR, *et al.* (2008) Motivation for contemporary tattoo removal. *Arch Dermatol* **144**: 879–884.
3. Anderson RR. (2001) Regarding tattoos. Is that sunlight or an oncoming train at the end of the tunnel? *Arch Dermatol* **137**: 210–212.

4. Laumann AE, Derick AJ. (2006) Tattoos and body piercings in the United States: a national data set. *J Am Acad Dermatol* **55**: 413–421.
5. Clabaugh W. (1968) Removal of tattoos by superficial dermabrasion. *Arch Dermatol* **98**: 515–521.
6. Colver GB, Dawber RP. (1984) Tattoo removal using a liquid nitrogen cryospray. *Clin Exp Dermatol* **9**: 364–366.
7. Bunke HJ, Conway H. (1957) Surgery of decorative and traumatic tattoos. *Plast Reconstr Surg* **20**: 67–69.
8. Bailin PL, Ratz JL, Levine HL. (1980) Removal of tattoos by CO_2 laser. *J Dermatol Surg Oncol* **6**: 997–1001.
9. Apfelberg DB, Maser MR, Lash H. (1979) Argon laser treatment of decorative tattoos. *Br J Plast Surg* **32**: 141–144.
10. Alster TS. (1995) Q-switched alexandrite laser treatment (755 nm) of professional and amateur tattoos. *J Am Acad Dermatol* **33**: 69–73.
11. Alster TS. (1995) Successful elimination of traumatic tattoos by the Q-switched alexandrite (755-nm) laser. *Ann Plast Surg* **34**: 542–545.
12. Grevelink JM, Duke D, van Leeuwen RL, *et al.* (1996) Laser treatment of tattoos in darkly pigmented patients: efficacy and side effects. *J Am Acad Dermatol* **34**: 653–656.
13. Goldstein N. (1987) Tattoo removal. *Dermatol Clin* **5**: 349–358.
14. Farber MG, Lamberg RL, Smith ME. (1986) A histologic study of eyelid pigment eight weeks after implantation (eyelid tattoo). *Arch Opthalmol* **104**: 1434–1435.
15. Goldstein AP. (1979) Histologic reactions in tattoos. *J Dermatol Surg Oncol* **5**: 896–900.
16. Dover JS, Margolis RJ, Polla LL, *et al.* (1989) Pigmented guinea pig skin irradiated with Q-switched ruby laser pulses. Morphologic and histologic findings. *Arch Dermatol* **125**: 43–49.
17. Anderson RR, Parrish JA. (1983) Selective photothermolysis: precise microsurgery by selective absorption of pulsed radiation. *Science* **220**: 524–527.
18. Kilmer SL. (1997) Laser treatment of tattoos. *Dermatol Clin* **15**: 409–417.
19. Ashinoff R, Geronemus RG. (1992) Rapid response of traumatic and medical tattoos to treatment with the Q-switched ruby laser. *Lasers Surg Med Suppl* **4**: 71.
20. Geronemus RG, Ashinoff R. (1991) Use of the Q-switched ruby laser to treat tattoos and benign pigmented lesions of the skin. *Lasers Surg Med Suppl* **3**: 64.
21. DeCoste SD, Anderson RR. (1991) Comparison of Q-switched ruby and Q-switched Nd:YAG laser treatment of tattoos. *Lasers Surg Med Suppl* **3**: 64.
22. Kilmer SL, Anderson RR. (1993) Clinical use of the Q-switched ruby and the Q-switched Nd:YAG (1064 nm and 532 nm) lasers for treatment of tattoos. *J Dermatol Surg Oncol* **19**: 330–338.
23. Fitzpatrick RE, Goldman MP, Ruiz-Esparza J. (1993) Use of the alexandrite laser (755 nm, 100 nsec) for tattoo pigment removal in an animal model. *J Am Acad Dermatol* **28**: 745–750.
24. Garcia C, Clark RE. (1995) Tattoo removal using the alexandrite laser. *N C Med J* **56**: 336–338.
25. Fitzpatrick RE, Goldman MP. (1994) Tattoo removal using the alexandrite laser. *Arch Dermatol* **130**: 1508–1514.
26. McMeekin TO, Goodwin DP. (1993) A comparison of the alexandrite laser (755 nm) with the Q-switched ruby laser (694 nm) in the treatment of tattoos. *Lasers Surg Med Suppl* **5**: 43.
27. Ferguson JE, August PJ. (1996) Evaluation of the Nd:YAG laser for treatment of amateur and professional tattoos. *Br J Dermatol* **135**: 586–591.
28. Jones A, Roddy P, Orengo I, *et al.* (1996) The Q-switched Nd:YAG laser effectively treats tattoos in darkly pigmented skin. *Dermatol Surg* **22**: 999–1001.
29. Kilmer SL, Lee M, Farinelli W, *et al.* (1992) Q-switched Nd: YAG laser (1064 nm) effectively treats Q-switched ruby laser resistant tattoos. *Lasers Surg Med Suppl* **4**: 72.
30. Kilmer SL, Lee MS, Grevelink JM, *et al.* (1993) The Q-switched Nd:YAG laser effectively treats tattoos. A controlled, dose-response study. *Arch Dermatol* **129**: 971–978.
31. Kilmer SL, Farinelli WF, Tearney G, *et al.* (1994) Use of a larger spot size for the treatment of tattoos increase clinical efficacy and decreases potential side effects. *Laser Surg Med Suppl* **6**: 51.
32. Kilmer SL, Lee MS, Anderson RR. (1993) Treatment of multi-colored tattoos with the Q-switched Nd:YAG laser (532 nm): a dose response study with comparison to the Q-switched ruby laser. *Lasers Surg Med Suppl* **5**: 54.
33. Kirby W, Desai A, Desai T. (2009) The Kirby-Desai Scale. A proposed scale to assess tattoo removal treatments. *J of Clin and Aesthetic Dermatology* **2**: 32–37.
34. Goldstein N. (1979) Complications from tattoos. *J Dermatol Surg Oncol* **5**: 869–878.
35. Lanigan SW. (2003) Incidence of side effects after laser hair removal. *J Am Acad Dermatol* **49**: 882–886.
36. Handley JM. (2006) Adverse events associated with nonblative cutaneous visible and infrared laser treatment. *J Am Acad Dermatol* **55**: 482–489.

37. Kilmer SL, Casparian JM, Wimberly JM, *et al.* (1993) Hazards of Q-switched lasers. *Lasers Surg Med Suppl* **5**: 56.
38. Anderson RR, Geronemus R, Kilmer SL, *et al.* (1993) Cosmetic tattoos ink darkening. A complication of Q-switched and pulsed-laser treatment. *Arch Dermatol* **129**: 1010–1014.
39. Ashinoff R, Levine VJ, Soter NA. (1995) Allergic reactions to tattoo pigment after laser treatment. *Dermatol Surg* **21**: 291–294.
40. Ballin DB. (1933) Cutaneous hypersensitivity to mercury from tattooing: report of case. *Arch Dermatol Syph* **27**: 292.
41. Bjornberg A. (1963) Reactions to light in yellow tattoos from cadmium sulphide. *Arch Dermatol* **88**: 267.
42. Bjornberg A. (1959) Allergic reactions to chrome in green tattoo markings. *Acta Derm Venereal* **39**: 23.
43. Dickinson JA. (1969) Sarcoidal reactions in tattoos. *Arch Dermatol* **100**: 315–319.
44. Yang DS, Kim SC, Lee S, *et al.* (1989) Foreign body epithelioid granuloma after cosmetic eyebrow tattooing. *Cutis* **43**: 244–247.

Chapter 7

Laser Hair Removal in the Asian Skin

Su-Ping Lim, Regina*

Introduction

Hair removal has been practised by both women and men for centuries. Hair removal methods have from prehistoric flint and copper razors developed to tweezing, threading, sugaring and waxing developed by the ancient cultures, to better techniques using Gillette razors in the 1900s, and later chemical depilation and electrolysis. The most significant and sophisticated advance has been the introduction of lasers for hair removal when the FDA approved in 1995, the first laser for hair removal. The desire for more effective and longer lasting hair reduction with minimal complication rates has led to a wide variety of lasers and broadband light sources being developed and marketed for hair removal. Asian skin is more susceptible to pigmentary and other side effects of laser hair removal, hence the choice of laser and technique of the operator are of paramount importance for a successful outcome as well as patient satisfaction.

Specific Qualities in Asian Hair and Skin

Asian hair has a larger diameter and is usually rounded and very straight as compared with other ethnic groups.[1] Whilst Asian hair follicles are thicker, the hair density is less compared with Caucasoid hair and Afrocarribean hair.[2] Asian hair has more eumelanin which imparts the darker brown black colors than phaeomelanin which imparts the red hues.[3,4] In skin, there is no evidence of racial differences in terms of the number of melanocytes and it is the variation in the numbers, size and aggregation of melanosomes within the melanocytes and keratinocytes that accounts for the differences in skin color between races. Asian skin shows mainly aggregated melanosomes in non-exposed sites of skin and predominantly non-aggregated melanosomes in sunlight-exposed skin.[5–7] Asians typically exhibit skin type III–V on the Fitzpatrick skin type scale. The darker skin types show a higher epidermal melanin content and a higher propensity to post-inflammatory hyperpigmentation.[5,8]

How Lasers Remove Hair

Lasers employ the principle of selective photothermolysis to remove hair. Using a specific wavelength of laser light allows for selective targeting of chromophores which preferentially absorbs this light with resultant thermal energy to destroy specific targets. In hair removal, the target chromophore is melanin and the target for destruction is the hair bulge section of the hair follicle.[9] Careful consideration of the wavelength, fluence, pulse duration, thermal relaxation time and competing chromophores is essential in maximizing the efficacy and minimizing the adverse events of the procedure.

Melanin absorbs in the optical window between 600–1100 nm, with decreased absorption at longer

*Consultant Dermatologist, Department of Dermatology, Changi General Hospital, Singapore.

wavelengths. The longer wavelengths, however, allow for deeper penetration of the laser light into the skin. Competing chromophores such as hemoglobin absorb poorly in this range. The presence of melanin within the epidermis (which is a competing site), is a cause of concern with epidermal injury and other adverse effects. In terms of the hair cycle, it is during the anagen phase that melanin production occurs and becomes part of the growing follicle; it is during the anagen phase that the laser energy can be utilized to damage the bulge.

The hair follicle is made up of three main regions the infundibulum, isthmus and hair bulb (Fig. 7.1). The important source of pluripotent stem cells is located in the hair bulge, which is sited approximately one third of the distance from the skin surface to the follicle bulb.[9]

For effective longer lasting hair removal, it is the hair bulge that needs to be damaged. The follicular stem cells in the bulge are not pigmented but pulses longer than the thermal relaxation time of the hair shaft will allow thermal energy to be propagated through the hair follicle to effect damage to the stem cells.[10] So a balance has to be struck for ideal laser pulse duration. For confinement of the thermal damage, the pulse duration should be shorter than or equal to the thermal relaxation time (TRT) of the hair follicle. Thermal damage time to allow for damage to the actual target of the hair bulge requires pulses longer than the thermal relaxation time of the hair follicle.[10] The thermal relaxation time of human hair follicles is estimated at about 10–100 ms.[11,12] Most current hair removal lasers have pulse durations in this millisecond range.

Another consideration of thermokinetic selectivity with pulse duration is that, with the same chromophore, a longer pulse duration allows for intrapulse cooling of smaller targets more rapidly than larger targets. Thus, if the thermal relaxation time of the basal layer (about 0.1 ms) or the epidermis (about 10 ms) is exceeded, then these smaller targets will cool more as they are heated through the laser pulse, hence the longer pulse duration actually selectively injures the

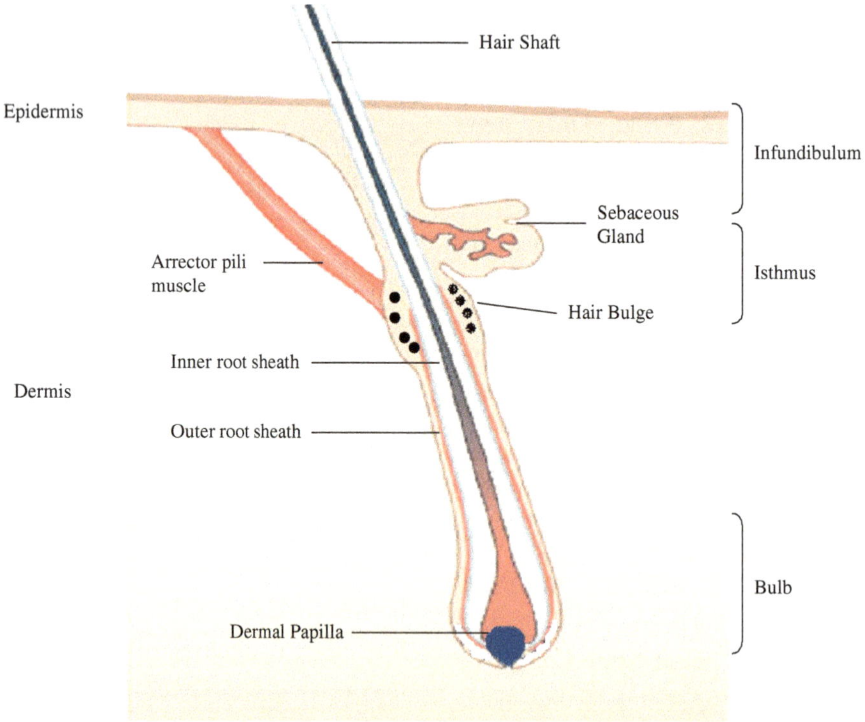

Figure 7.1.

Diagram of a hair follicle showing the position of the hair bulge.

hair follicles whilst sparing the smaller targets in the epidermis.[13]

Fluence (energy density measured in J/cm^2) is an important factor in the efficacy of the procedure but is limited by how much the patient can tolerate safely.[14,15] This limiting factor is determined largely by skin color. The fluence required for coagulation of the hair follicle is proportional to the shaft diameter: the thicker the hair diameter, the higher the fluence level required.[16] Asian hair has a larger diameter compared with other skin types but also contains large amounts of eumelanin that more readily absorbs the energy as compared with phaeomelanin: to some extent this compensates for and reduces the fluence required for effective hair removal.

For therapeutic ease and efficiency, the spot size selected would ideally be as large as possible to reduce scattering of the light as well as reducing the time required for the treatment procedure.[17]

Considering all the variables that influence the choice of lasers, for the Asian patient, the use of longer wavelengths would in theory increase the ratio of energy deposited in the dermis to that in the epidermis, which should better injure the bulge through heating with epidermal sparing. Also, longer wavelengths result in less absorption by melanin that is present in the epidermis. Longer pulse durations would be safer for darker skin types, according to the theory of thermokinetic selectivity,[13] but too long a pulse duration, i.e. exceeding the TRT of the hair follicle, would result in loss of confinement of the thermal damage to the hair follicle and would conversely result in thermal injury to non-follicular structures.

Laser Selection

There are many systems in use today for laser hair removal. These include the ruby laser (694 nm), alexandrite (755 nm), diode (800–1000 nm) and long-pulsed neodymium yttrium-aluminum-garnet (Nd:YAG) (1064 nm), as well as intense pulsed light (IPL) (550–1200 nm) sources. This section will include a brief description of these lasers available commercially, with emphasis on the safer options in Asian skin.

Long-pulsed 1064 nm Nd:YAG Lasers

The longer wavelength utilized in this laser system penetrates deeply. The poor absorption by epidermal melanin at this wavelength makes this one of the safest options in darker skin types. Additional cooling devices within these systems also protect the epidermis. However, the poorer absorption by melanin at 1064 nm also means that higher fluences and possibly more treatment sessions are required to effect hair removal.

Commercial systems using this long pulsed wavelength include the CoolGlide™ (Cutera), Lyra/Gemini™ (Laserscope), Ultrawave™ (Adept Medical), Athos™ (Quantel), GentleYAG™ (Candela), Profile™ (Sciton), VascuLight™ (Lumenis), SmartEpill™ and Acclaim™ (Cyanosure), Dualis™ (Fotona), Varia™ (CoolTouch) and Mydon™ (Wavelight). The Coolglide™ and Lyra/Gemini™ systems utilizes contact precooling and contact cooling respectively, the GentleYAG™ has a cryogen spray and the Ultrawave™ has a photon recycling system. The various systems have varying capabilities in terms of pulse duration, fluence and repetition rates and information on these are readily available from the manufacturers.

Diode Laser 800–1000 nm

With the longer wavelength, additional active cooling and longer pulse durations, the diode laser is also suitable for darker skin types. Commercial systems include the LightSheer™ (Lumenis), Apex-800™ (Iridex), SLP1000™ (Palomar), MedioStar™ (Aesclepion-Meditec), F1 Diode Laser™ (Opusmed) and EpiStar™ (Nidek).

Long-pulsed Alexandrite Laser 755 nm

The long-pulsed alexandrite laser has also been shown to be safe for darker skin types, provided great care, precautions and cooling measures are taken as more complications can occur with this shorter wavelength system. Commercial systems in use include the Apogee™ (Cyanosure), Epitouch Alex™ (Lumenis), GentleLase™ (Candela), Ultrawave II–III™ (Adept Medical) and Epicare™ (LightAge). The Ultrawave II–III™ also includes the 1064 nm wavelength capability in a single device.

Long-pulsed Ruby Laser 694 nm

With the shortest wavelength of the laser hair removal systems, the long-pulsed ruby laser is less suitable for darker skin types as the risk of adverse effects such as hyper- and hypopigmentation and scarring is higher as compared with the longer wavelength devices. Commercial long-pulsed ruby lasers in use include Ruby Star™ (Aesclepion-Meditec), Sinon™ (Wavelight), E2000™ (Palomar), Epitouch Ruby™ (Sharplan) and Chromos™ (Mehl Biophile).

Intense Pulsed Light (IPL) Systems

Intense pulsed broadband light sources have also been used for hair removal. Using filters gives the option of wavelength selection, and the wide choices of wavelength, pulse duration and pulse modes/intervals allow the potential for different skin types to be treated effectively. Many of these devices are user friendly, with software programs to guide treatment parameter selection according to the skin type, hair color and texture. Commercially available systems include the Epilight™ (Lumenis), Quantum HR™ (Lumenis), Ellipse™ (DDD), Photolight™ (Cyanosure), Estelux™ (Palomar), ProLite™ (Alderm), Spatouch™ (Radiancy), Quadra Q4™ (Derma Med USA) and SpectraPulse™ (Primary Technology). Some companies have also developed combination systems with IPL and Nd:YAG available in a single device like the VascuLight™ (Lumenis) and Starlux™ (Palomar).

Comparison of Efficacy and Adverse Effects between the Laser Systems

With the wide variety of laser and IPL systems available, choosing the right system to minimize side effects for the Asian patient is important. There are studies comparing the efficacy of the different laser systems but as responses to laser hair removal vary considerably between patients, depending on the skin type, hair color, anatomical site and treatment intervals, definitive conclusions are difficult. This point is highlighted with differing conclusions drawn in studies on efficacy. The alexandrite laser was found to be more efficacious as compared with the Nd:YAG laser in some studies.[18,19] Yet others have found no significant differences between them.[20,21]

Previous studies have reported on the incidence of side effects. These have involved relatively few treatment episodes and patients.[22,23] One of the largest studies to date is a multicenter prospective study of 480 patients receiving 3143 treatments in the United Kingdom, assessing the incidence of side effects in relation to skin type and lasers used.[24] Laser hair removal procedures were carried out by both doctors and trained nurses following protocols, and lasers used in the study included the long-pulsed ruby, long-pulsed alexandrite and long-pulsed Nd:YAG. Epidermal cooling devices such as gels, cold air, cryogen spray or cold contact plates were used as appropriate. A three-month study period assessed all the patients undergoing laser hair removal who had at least one previous laser treatment for side effects. Of 3143 treatments, 322 treatments utilized the ruby laser, 74 utilized the alexandrite and 224 utilized the Nd:YAG.

For skin types I–II, the ruby laser was used in 191 patients, producing blistering in 13 (6%). The alexandrite laser was used in 50 patients and blistering occurred in 1 (2%). The Nd:YAG laser was used in 92 patients and blistering was seen in 2 (2%). Hypopigmentation with the ruby laser was 1.6% and hyperpigmentation 1%.

For skin type III, the incidence of blistering with the ruby laser was 4.5%; with the alexandrite laser, 0%; and with the Nd:YAG laser, 8.8%. The incidence of hyperpigmentation, with the ruby laser was 2.8%; alexandrite laser, 0%; and the Nd:YAG laser, 3%. Hypopigmentation occurred in only one patient following Nd:YAG laser therapy.

For patients with skin type IV–VI (109 patients in total), the incidence of blistering with the ruby laser was 14.9% and with the Nd:YAG laser, 5%. The incidence of hyperpigmentation with the ruby laser was 9.9% as compared with 2.1% with the Nd:YAG laser. The overall incidence of side effects for this group was 9.4% with the Nd:YAG laser and 29.9% with the ruby laser.

In addition, the study also recorded atrophic scarring in one patient with skin type III following treatment with the ruby laser on the face. This scarring eventually almost cleared and further treatment in the same patient later did not result in any further sequelae. One case of superficial thrombophlebitis also developed on the chin following treatment with the ruby and Nd:YAG lasers, persisting for one week.

This large prospective study has shown a very low incidence of persistent side effects. It also confirms that increased incidence of side effects is seen in darker skin types, particularly where treatment with the ruby laser is carried out. The recommendation from the study is that the ruby laser should not be used in darker skin types when alternatives such as the Nd:YAG laser can be used more safely.

Ruby Laser

In a Scandinavian study using the ruby laser, Bjerring *et al.*[25] reviewed 133 patients and reported 14.3% experiencing hyperpigmentation and 9.8% experiencing hypopigmentation. The study by Sommer *et al.*[22] reported erythema and swelling in 61% and blistering in 14%. Minor crusting was seen in 33%. All resolved within two to three days. Mild hyperpigmentation (17%) resolved within six months and hypopigmentation was not seen. Permanent textural skin changes or scarring were not seen. Wimmershoff *et al.*[26] in a study of 74 patients, reported hyperpigmentation in 5%, hypopigmentation in 3% and atrophic scarring in 3%, with scarring occurring only in darker skin types. All the patients with hypopigmentary changes had skin types III to IV.

Alexandrite Laser

With the alexandrite laser studies, Nanni and Alster[27] reported blistering and/or fine epidermal crusting in 10–15% of patients and significantly more so in darker skin types but long term complications and scarring were rare.[28,29]

Eremia *et al.*[30] in a study of 89 untanned patients with skin types I–IV undergoing 492 treatments, reported complications limited to transient post-inflammatory hyperpigmentation in 10% and post-inflammatory hypopigmentation in 2%, with one patient experiencing a burn with blistering. No scarring was noted. Another study from Saudi Arabia[23] on 150 patients with skin type IV–VI reported complications in 2.7% of body locations, showing axillary and bikini areas to be at risk. Two patients with skin type VI had adverse reactions with severe blistering seen in one. The authors also commented that residual pigmentary changes were seen in this skin type. Paradoxical hypertrichosis was first reported with intense pulsed light therapy.[31] This has also been reported with alexandrite laser treatment.[32] A possible explanation of this unusual phenomenon is that the suboptimal fluences used may be too low to cause thermolysis of the hair follicles but produce enough energy to create a heat shock that conversely induces follicular stem cell differentiation and growth.[33,34]

Contributing factors to paradoxical hypertrichosis include darker skin types (III–VI), sites (face and neck, in particular the mandibular area and the chin), suboptimal treatment fluences and the presence of untreated hormonal influences (e.g. polycystic ovarian syndrome).[32,33] Treatment to address paradoxical hypertrichosis include the use of higher fluences as well as cold packs or wet gauze to prevent heat diffusion to untreated areas.[33] A large Turkish study of 2359 patients showed a complication rate of 2.2% using the long-pulsed alexandrite laser in patients with skin types II–V, with pigmentary changes, folliculitis and blistering being the most common complications.[35] Another study using the alexandrite laser on 144 Asian subjects with skin types III–V showed that the use of this laser in Asian skin required great caution as consistent safety was not noted.[36] Figure 7.2 illustrates the presence of crusting after alexandrite laser hair removal.

Diode and Nd:YAG Lasers

A number of studies have demonstrated the efficacy of longer wavelength devices such as the diode and Nd:YAG lasers in hair removal[19,37–40] and that they are efficacious in patients with darker skin types.[41,42] In a study comparing the long-pulsed diode and long-pulsed alexandrite laser, patients rated intra- and postoperative pain with the alexandrite laser as being mild to moderate as compared with the diode, for which the patients rated the pain as moderate to severe especially at higher fluences.[38] Transient hyperpigmentation was seen in 10% with the diode laser. There was no evidence of scarring or atrophy.

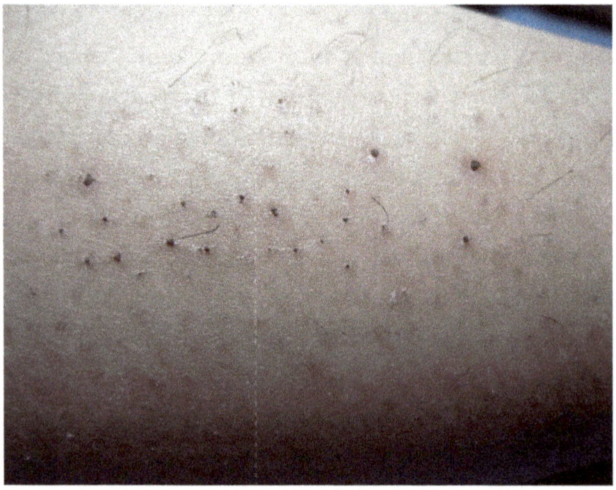

Figure 7.2.

Fine crusting seen a few days after alexandrite laser hair removal on a small test area.

In one study of the long-pulsed Nd:YAG laser for hair removal, complete depilation was reported after 4–6 sessions in 208 patients, with no blistering or pigmentary changes.[39] These results have not been matched in subsequent studies. Another study investigated 20 patients with skin types IV–VI treated with the long-pulsed Nd:YAG.[42] Adverse effects were limited to mild to moderate pain at 90% of treatment sites; transient pigmentary alterations in 5% affecting exposed facial and leg areas only; and vesiculation in 1.5%. Fibrosis or scarring was not seen. Histological tissue changes mirrored the clinical response rates with evidence of selective follicular injury without epidermal disruption. Again, paradoxical hair growth induced by diode laser therapy has been reported.[43]

A recently reported side effect is reticulate erythema following diode laser hair removal.[44]

IPL Systems

Studies have also confirmed the efficacy of IPL systems for hair removal.[45,46] One of these studies[46] compared the long and short-pulsed alexandrite laser with the IPL system, and found no statistically significant difference in efficacy. Transient side effects were highest in the long-pulsed alexandrite group and least in the IPL system. Another study found mild and reversible side effects with the IPL system in a minority of patients (hyperpigmentation in 9%, superficial crusting in 6%) using wavelengths of 615–695 nm.[45] A study of 49 patients undergoing 390 treatment sessions of IPL photodepilation reported transient erythema ($n = 30$); late evanescent erythema ($n = 3$); mild pain ($n = 43$); moderate pain ($n = 6$); crust formation ($n = 9$); superficial burning ($n = 1$); isolated vesicles ($n = 3$); transient hyperpigmentation ($n = 8$); transient hypopigmentation ($n = 1$); persistent heat sensation locally ($n = 1$); and minimal scar ($n = 1$).[31] This study also reported the paradoxical effect of the growth of new fine, dark hair in five patients involving untreated areas in close proximity to the treated areas, suggesting that intense pulsed light may induce activation of dormant hair follicles in untreated areas close to hirsute-treated areas. This unusual side effect of paradoxical hair growth has also been reported in other cases where IPL systems were used for other indications such as the treatment of port-wine stains.[47] This side effect has now been reported with IPL, long-pulsed alexandrite, diode and Nd:YAG lasers and is likely to be common to all the current light and laser hair removal devices. Temporary or permanent leukotrichia can also develop following IPL hair removal. In a study of 821 patients, 29 treated patients developed leukotrichia with restoration of color only occurring in nine patients within two to six months.[48] A Singapore study compared single treatment responses to the long-pulsed Nd:YAG laser and IPL therapy for hair removal in skin types IV–VI.[49] Patients were treated on one half of the body with the long-pulsed Nd:YAG and the other half with the IPL system. Patients found the pain from the two systems different, but both tolerable. Greater efficacy was seen with the Nd:YAG laser. Post-inflammatory hyperpigmentation occurred in some patients with the IPL treated sides but not the Nd:YAG laser treated sides, with three patients experiencing blistering followed by post-inflammatory hyperpigmentation. The author found that the long-pulsed Nd:YAG produced sufficient follicular injury with less epidermal damage in patients with darker skin types as compared with the shorter wavelength light system.

Data from these studies may be influenced by the tendency to select lasers for patients according to their skin types, while the small numbers of patients in some studies may also not reflect the true incidence of side effects. Table 7.1 shows the time frames associated with the adverse effects. It is important to bear in mind that these are fairly uncommon and short-lived, with a very low incidence of permanent sequelae. We advocate the use of longer wavelength lasers such as the Nd:YAG for patients with darker skin types to further reduce the risk of side effects. Guidelines for photoepilation are also available to laser practitioners.[50,51]

Table 7.1.

Principal Adverse Effects of Laser/IPL Hair Removal

Principal Adverse Effects of Laser/IPL Hair Removal
Acute short-term effects (lasting hours to days)
Pain
Perifollicular erythema
Edema
Blistering
Crusting
Folliculitis
Purpura
Thrombophlebitis
Cold urticaria
Post-inflammatory transient effects (lasting weeks to months)
Hyperpigmentation
Hypopigmentation
Leukotrichia
Reticulate erythema
Permanent adverse effects (rare)
Hyperpigmentation
Hypopigmentation
Atrophy
Scarring
Leukotrichia
Paradoxical hypertrichosis (?permanent)

Patient Care Before, During and After Treatment

It is important before performance of laser hair removal on any patient to take a thorough history, examine the patient and assess the individual's benefit and risk potential. It is prudent to counsel the patient carefully and obtain written informed consent before proceeding with the treatment.

Pre-treatment photographs may be taken as an option, again with consent.

Pre-treatment Assessment

History

- Site and duration of problem. Quality of life impact.
- Present hair removal techniques and previous techniques used. Any side effects experienced with such techniques.
- Any history of previous treatment with lasers/IPL for hair removal and any side effects experienced.
- Patient expectations.
- Any co-existing medical problems, e.g. polycystic ovarian syndrome (PCOS), acne, folliculitis, adrenal and other tumors, herpes simplex, bleeding dyscrasias, photosensitive dermatoses, koebnerizing dermatoses like vitiligo, psoriasis, lichen planus.
- Drug history: drugs causing hirsutism/hypertrichosis, photosensitizing drugs, drugs predisposing to poor healing (e.g. systemic steroids or bleeding risks), oral isotretinoin within one year, gold therapy (risk of localized chrysiasis).
- Scarring and pigmentary history.
- Previous tattoos.
- Tanning history, occupation, recent holidays, photoprotective practices.

Examination

- Site.
- Hair thickness, density, color.
- Skin type.
- Pigmentary or scarring changes.
- Presence within treatment site of tattoos or nevi.
- Any signs of other medical problems.

If the patient is suitable for treatment and is capable of understanding the risks and has realistic expectations, then proceed to careful counselling with clear explanation of the procedure and risks, and obtain written informed consent.

Pre-treatment Advice to Patient

- Avoid sun tan and use sunblock regularly. If tanned recently, postpone treatment for at least 6–8 weeks and practise sun protection to fade tan.
- Avoid plucking, waxing, tweezing, threading and using hair bleaching creams. Shave only if required and shave 1–2 days prior to the procedure. Hair depilatory creams may be used as an alternative.
- Administer prophylactic oral antiviral treatment (e.g. aciclovir) if necessary for patients prone to herpes simplex infections, 1–2 days prior to treatment.
- Administer prophylactic oral antibiotic treatment (e.g. anti-Staphylococcal antibiotics) for patients prone to recurrent folliculitis 1–2 days prior to treatment.
- Prophylactic oral treatment may be given for 5–7 days as indicated.

Pre-treatment Preparation for the Day

- Ensure hair is short enough for procedure (not more than 1–2 mm off skin surface) and no active infection in treatment site. Clip/shave if necessary.
- Clean treatment area and remove all makeup.
- Apply topical anesthesia (e.g. EMLA®, Astra Zeneca) one hour prior to the procedure.
- Clean topical anesthesia off and apply cooled gel to facilitate cooling of the skin and glide of laser if applicable.
- Laser protective goggles for patient and staff in attendance.

Treatment Technique

Ideal treatment parameters are individualized according to the patient, and treatment protocols can

Table 7.2.

Example of a Treatment Protocol for Asian Patients Using Coolglide™ Long-pulsed Nd:YAG 1064 nm Laser

10 mm spot size
1–2 Hz repetition rate
Adequate pre-parallel- and post-cooling
Optional: Test areas
Fluence: increase by approximately 5–10% with successive treatment if well tolerated. Maintain if good response with adequate endpoints.

Fitzpatrick Skin Type	Site	Fluence (J/cm^2)	Pulse Duration (ms)
III/IV	Face	35–50	20
	Non-facial	40–55	20
V/VI	Face	30–45	30
	Non-facial	35–50	30

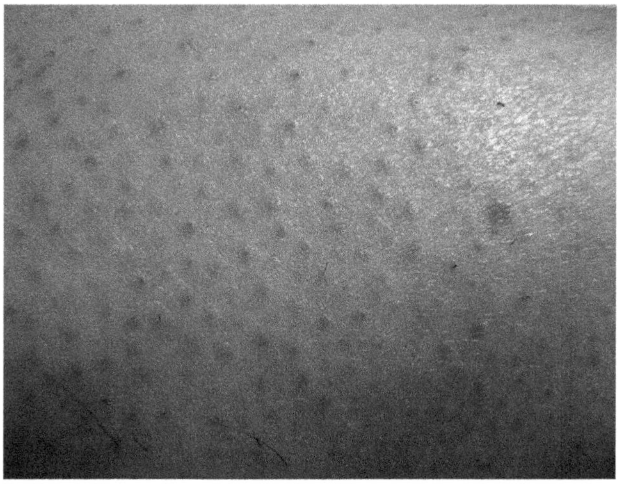

Figure 7.3.

Expected endpoint of perifollicular edema and mild erythema minutes after laser hair removal.

be used as a guide (Table 7.2). If necessary, test spots may be carried out on inconspicuous areas. Careful attention needs to be paid to prevent double treatment and missed areas. The use of cooled gel helps guide the operator with the gel forming gridlines during treatment. The skin needs to be closely observed for any immediate signs of acute epidermal injury like whitening/graying, blistering or erosions. The laser is held perpendicular to the skin surface with gentle pressure against the skin, and slightly overlapping pulses should be delivered with checking of the treated skin regularly for expected endpoints or any unwanted immediate adverse effects. The individual laser systems have specific pre-treatment, parallel-treatment and post-treatment cooling measures which should be employed to protect the epidermis (e.g. pre-treatment cryogen spurts, cooling gel, contact cooling hand pieces, continuous flow of chilled air).

The expected endpoint is the immediate vaporization of the hair shaft, followed by perifollicular edema and mild erythema minutes later (Fig. 7.3), without any evidence of acute epidermal injury.

Resulting from vaporization of the hair follicles, the unpleasant sulfuric smell of the laser plume may be removed by the use of a smoke evacuator. After completion of the procedure, ensure the laser machine is put back on a standby mode before removal of protective eye goggles. The clinic notes should be clearly documented to include the laser parameters used, endpoints seen and details of the procedure such as preoperative measures, patient's tolerance of the actual procedure and postoperative measures and advice.

Postoperative Care and Advice

Cooling measures such as ice packs, cold rollers and aloe vera gel can be used to reduce postoperative pain and minimize swelling. Analgesics are rarely required unless large areas are treated. A topical antibiotic ointment may be used if there is any epidermal injury. Any prophylactic antiviral or antibiotic treatment courses should be completed. The patient should avoid picking or scratching the area. Sun avoidance advice should be reiterated. The patient should also be told regarding what to expect with hair casts shedding which typically occurs during the first week post-procedure as well as be reassured this is not new hair growth. Make up should be avoided until 48 hours post-procedure or until any blistering/crusts fully resolve.

Follow-up Treatments

The follow-up treatment intervals are usually between six to eight weeks. Treatment can be repeated when regrowth occurs, and this is dependent on the hair cycle which does vary according to the anatomic site. Therefore, a six-week interval is more typical for facial sites and an eight-week interval for the trunk and limbs.

Case Studies

Case 1

A 40-year-old Chinese female with skin type IV was seen for laser removal of the hairs on her upper lip and lower legs. She was well with no significant medical history of note. Previous treatments included depilatory creams, waxing and shaving. She received six treatments at six-weekly intervals to the upper lip area with a Coolglide™ Nd:YAG 1064 nm laser (gradual increments from 36–42 J/cm², 20 ms pulse duration, 10 mm spot size) with 80% hair reduction, good patient satisfaction and no side effects. As for her legs, she received six treatments with the same laser at eight-weekly intervals (gradual increments from 38–40 J/cm², 20 ms pulse duration, 10 mm spot size) (Fig. 7.4).

Again there was good hair reduction of 80%. There was some mild transient hyperpigmentation around the hair follicles (Fig. 7.5) which resolved post-treatment within weeks without intervention.

Case 2

A 30-year-old Chinese male consulted regarding laser hair removal of chest and abdominal hairs. He has skin type IV and is well with no medical history of note. Previous hair removal techniques had included shaving and one previous laser hair removal at another clinic.

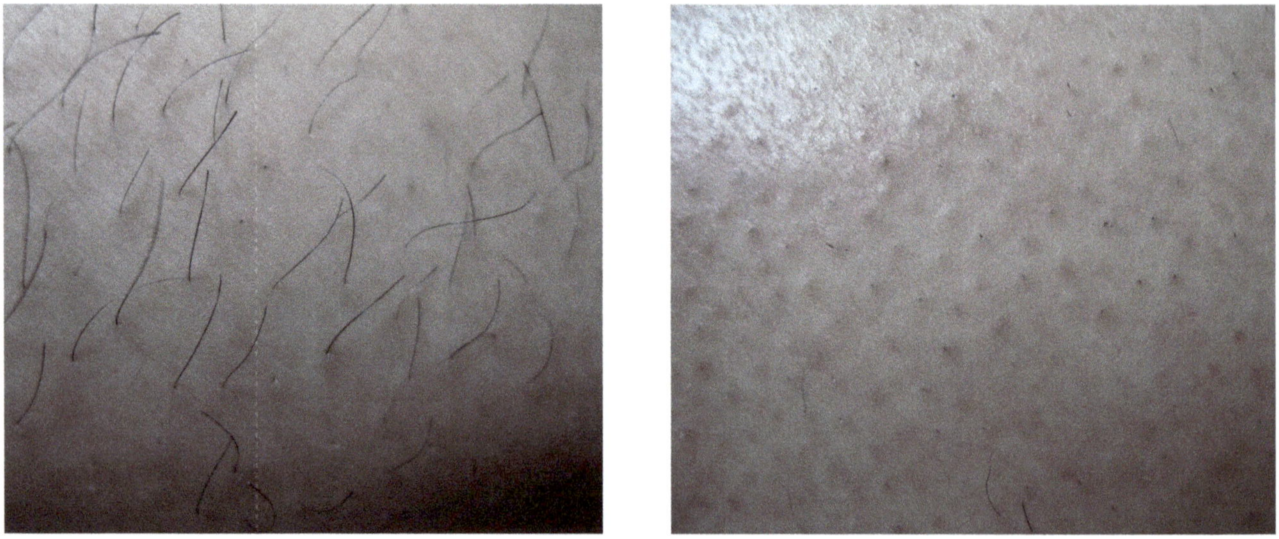

(a) (b)

Figure 7.4.

(a) Before laser hair removal (legs). (b) After one session of long-pulsed 1064 nm Nd:YAG laser hair removal.

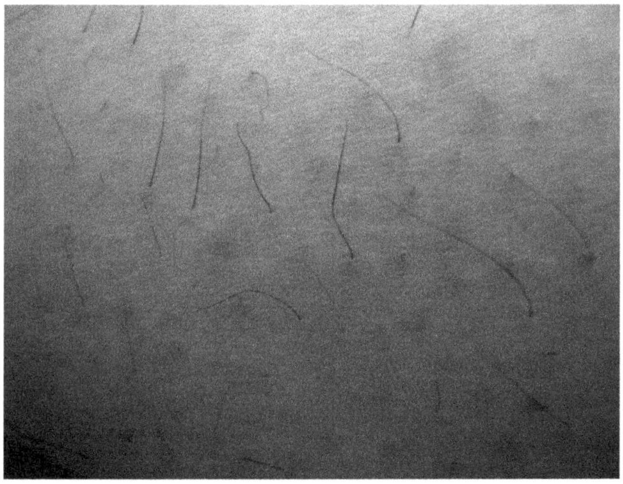

Figure 7.5.

Mild transient perifollicular hyperpigmentation which resolved spontaneously within weeks.

Treatment with the Coolglide™ Nd:YAG 1064 nm laser was carried out at 6–8 weekly intervals and the patient had completed a series of six treatments at 50 J/cm^2, 20 ms pulse duration, 10 mm spot size, with 90% reduction in hairs. Treatment was well tolerated with no side effects.

Case 3

A 29-year-old Indian female, skin type V consulted regarding axillary hair removal. She had a tendency to post-inflammatory pigmentation problems but was otherwise fit and well. A test area was initially carried out using the Coolglide™ Nd:YAG laser 1064 nm with fluence of 35 J/cm^2, a longer pulse duration of 30 ms and 10 mm spot size. There were no problems tolerating this fluence and she underwent six treatments at 6–8 weekly intervals tolerating all the treatments well with good hair reduction of more than 80%. She was prepared to accept that the thin finer hairs would not be removed and happy not to have the fluence increased further in view of her previous history of problems with post-inflammatory hyperpigmentation.

Recent Progress and Developments in Laser Hair Removal

With any laser technology, there are constant efforts to improve efficacy, reduce side effects and improve ease of treatment.

Pneumatic skin flattening devices have been developed to control pain associated with laser hair removal.[52] A new FDA approved Photopneumatic Therapy™ (Aesthera Corp, Livermore CA) combines broadband light with pneumatic energy to elevate the hair follicle closer to the surface of the skin to improve efficiency.[53,54]

Topical eflornithine HCL, Vaniqa® (Bristol Myers Squibb, Canada) is a recent introduction to aid removal and reduce the regrowth of unwanted facial hair. This has been used successfully in combination with lasers to improve hair removal, especially of the more laser resistant white or light colored hairs.[55]

It has also been the aim of laser and IPL companies to develop home-use devices for hair removal.[56] It remains to be seen whether these devices are safe enough or effective enough for mass consumer use, with the main issues being adequate safety measures to prevent treatment on sun-tanned skin and on the appropriate skin tone at the energy levels required for efficacy. Eye safety is an additional important concern.[56]

References

1. Franbourg A, Hallegot P, Baltenneck F, *et al.* (2003) Current research on ethnic hair. *J Am Acad Dermatol* **48**(Suppl. 6): S115–S119.
2. Lee HJ, Ha SJ, Lee JH, *et al.* (2002) Hair counts from scalp biopsy specimens in Asians. *J Am Acad Dermatol* **46**: 218–221.
3. Suzuki I, Im S, Tada A, *et al.* (1999) Participation of the melanocortin-1 receptor in the UV control of pigmentation. *J Invest Dermatol Symp Proc* **4**: 29–34.

4. Hunt G, Kyne S, Ito S, *et al.* (1995) A. Eumelanin and phaeomelanin contents of human epidermis and cultured melanocytes. *Pigment Cell Res* **8**: 202–208.
5. Taylor SC. (2002) Skin of color: biology, structure, function, and implications for dermatologic disease. *J Am Acad Dermatol* **46**: S41–S62.
6. Olson RL, Gaylor J, Everett MA. (1973) Skin color, melanin, and erythema. *Arch Dermatol* **108**: 541–544.
7. Toda K, Patnak MK, Parrish A, *et al.* (1972) Alteration of racial differences in melanosome distribution in human epidermis after exposure to ultraviolet light. *Nat New Biol* **236**: 143–144.
8. Smit NPM, Kolb RM, Lentjes EGWM, *et al.* (1998) Variations in melanin formation by cultured melanocytes from different skin types. *Arch Dermatol Res* **290**: 342–349.
9. Sun TT, Costsarelis G, Lavker RM. (1991) Hair follicular stem cells: the bulge-activation hypothesis. *J Invest Dermatol* **96**: 77–78.
10. Altshuler GB, Anderson RR, Manstein D, *et al.* (2001) Extended theory of selective photothermolysis. *Lasers Surg Med* **29**: 416–432.
11. Anderson RR, Parrish JA. (1983) Selective photothermolysis: precise microsurgery by selective absorption of pulsed radiation. *Science* **220**: 524–527.
12. Van Gemert MJC, Welch AJ. (1989) Time constants in thermal laser medicine. *Lasers Surg Med* **9**: 405–421.
13. Ross EV, Ladin Z, Kreindel M, *et al.* (1999) Theoretical considerations in laser hair removal. *Dermatol Clin* **17**: 333–355.
14. Rogachefsky AS, Becker K, Weiss G, *et al.* (2002) Evaluation of a long-pulsed Nd:YAG laser at different parameters: an analysis of both fluence and pulse duration. *Dermatol Surg* **28**: 932–935.
15. Kato T, Omi T, Naito Z, *et al.* (2004) Histological hair removal study by ruby or alexandrite laser with comparative study on the effects of wavelength and fluence. *J Cosmet Laser Ther* **6**: 32–37.
16. Nestor MS. (1998) Laser hair removal: clinical results and practical applications of selective photothermolysis. *Skin Aging* **10**: 34–39.
17. Lask G, Eckhouse S, Slatkin M, *et al.* (1999) The role of laser and intense light source in photoepilation: a comparative evaluation. *J Cutan Laser Ther* **1**: 3–13.
18. Bouzari N, Tabatabai H, Abbasi Z, *et al.* (2004) Laser hair removal: comparison of long pulsed Nd:YAG, long pulsed alexandrite, and long pulsed diode lasers. *Dermatol Surg* **30**: 498–502.
19. Tanzi EL, Alster TS. (2004) Long pulsed 1064 nm Nd:YAG laser assisted hair removal in all skin types. *Dermatol Surg* **30**: 13–17.
20. Rao J, Goldman MP. (2005) Prospective, comparative evaluation of three laser systems used individually and in combination for axillary hair removal. *Dermatol Surg* **31**: 1671–1676.
21. Davoudi SM, Behnia F, Gorouhi F, *et al.* (2008) Comparison of long-pulsed alexandrite and Nd:YAG lasers, individually and in combination, for leg hair removal. *Arch Dermatol* **144**: 1323–1327.
22. Sommer S, Render C, Burd R, *et al.* (1998) Ruby laser treatment for hirsutism: clinical response and patient tolerance. *Br J Dermatol* **138**: 1009–1014.
23. Garcia C, Alamoudi H, Nakib M, *et al.* (2000) Alexandrite laser hair removal is safe for Fitzpatrick skin types IV–VI. *Dermatol Surg* **26**: 130–134.
24. Lanigan SW. (2003) Incidence of side effects after laser hair removal. *J Am Acad Dermatol* **49**: 882–886.
25. Bjerring P, Zachariae H, Lybecker H, *et al.* (1998) Evaluation of the free-running ruby laser for hair removal: a retrospective study. *Acta Derm Venereol (Stockh)* **78**: 48–51.
26. Wimmershoff MB, Scherer K, Lorenz S, *et al.* (2000) Hair removal using a 5-msec long pulsed ruby laser. *Dermatol Surg* **26**: 205–209.
27. Nanni CA, Alster TS. (1998) A practical review of laser-assisted hair removal using the Q-switched Nd:YAG, long-pulsed ruby and long-pulsed alexandrite lasers. *Dermatol Surg* **24**: 1399–1405.
28. Nanni CA, Alster TS. (1998) Efficacy of multiple hair removal sessions using the Q-switched Nd:YAG, long-pulsed ruby and long-pulsed alexandrite laser systems. *Lasers Surg Med* **22**(Suppl. 10): 40.
29. Nanni CA, Alster TS. (1998) Complications of laser-assisted hair removal using the Q-switched Nd:YAG, long-pulsed ruby and long-pulsed alexandrite lasers. *Lasers Surg Med* **22**(Suppl 10): 67.
30. Eremia S, Li CY, Umar SH, *et al.* (2001) Laser hair removal: long-term results with a 755 nm alexandrite laser. *Dermatol Surg* **27**: 920–924.
31. Moreno-Arias GA, Costelo-Branco C, Ferrando J. (2002) Side-effects after IPL photodepilation. *Dermatol Surg* **28**: 1131–1134.
32. Alajlan A, Shapiro J, Rivers JK, *et al.* (2005) Paradoxical hypertrichosis after laser epilation. *J Am Acad Dermatol* **53**: 85–88.

33. Desai S, Mahmoud BH, Bhatia AC, *et al.* (2010) Paradoxical hypertrichosis after laser therapy: a review. *Dermatol Surg* **36**: 291–298.
34. Bouzari N, Firooz AR. (2006) Lasers may induce terminal hair growth. *Dermatol Surg* **32**: 460.
35. Kutlubay Z. (2009) Alexandrite laser hair removal results in 2359 patients: a Turkish experience. *J Cosmet Laser Ther* **11**: 85–93.
36. Hussain M, Polnikorn N, Goldberng DJ. (2003) Laser-assisted hair removal in Asian skin: efficacy, complications, and the effect of single versus multiple treatments. *Dermatol Surg* **29**: 249–254.
37. Lou WW, Quintana AT, Geronemus RG, *et al.* (2000) Prospective study of hair reduction by diode laser (800 nm) with long term follow up. *Dermatol Surg* **26**: 428–432.
38. Handrick C, Alster TS. (2001) Comparison of long-pulsed diode and long-pulsed alexandrite lasers for hair removal: a long-term clinical and histologic study. *Dermatol Surg* **27**: 622–626.
39. Bencini PL, Luci A, Galimberti M, *et al.* (1999) Long-term epilation with long-pulsed neodymium: YAG laser. *Dermatol Surg* **25**: 175–178.
40. Goldberg DJ, Samady JA. (2000) Evaluation of a long-pulse Q-switched Nd:YAG laser for hair removal. *Dermatol Surg* **26**: 109–113.
41. Greppi I. (2001) Diode laser hair removal of the black patient. *Lasers Surg Med* **28**: 150–155.
42. Alster TS, Bryan H, Williams CM. (2001) Long-pulsed Nd:YAG laser-assisted hair removal in pigmented skin: a clinical and histological evaluation. *Arch Dermatol* **137**: 885–889.
43. Bernstein EF. (2005) Hair growth induced by diode laser treatment. *Dermatol Surg* **31**: 584–586.
44. Lapidoth M, Shafirstein G, Ben Amitai D, *et al.* (2004) Reticulate erythema following diode laser-assisted hair removal: a new side effect of a common procedure. *J Am Acad Dermatol* **51**: 774–777.
45. Sadick NS, Weiss RA, Shea CR, *et al.* (2000) Long-term photoepilation using a broad-spectrum intense pulsed light source. *Arch Dermatol* **136**: 1336–1340.
46. Marayiannis KB, Vlachos SP, Savva MP, *et al.* (2003) Efficacy of long and short pulse alexandrite lasers compared with an intense pulsed light source for epilation: a study on 532 sites in 389 patients. *J Cosmet Laser Ther* **5**: 140–145.
47. Vlachos SP, Kontoes PP. (2002) Development of terminal hair following skin lesion treatments with an intense pulsed light source. *Aesthetic Plast Surg* **26**: 303–307.
48. Radmanesh M, Mostaghimi M, Yousefi I, *et al.* (2002) Leukotrichia developed following application of intense pulsed light for hair removal. *Dermatol Surg* **28**: 572–574.
49. Goh CL. (2003) Comparative study on a single treatment response to long pulse Nd:YAG lasers and intense pulse light therapy for hair removal on skin type IV to VI — is longer wavelengths lasers preferred over shorter wavelengths lights for assisted hair removal. *J Dermatol Treat* **14**: 243–247.
50. Casey AS, Goldberg D. (2008) Guidelines for laser hair removal. *J Cosmet Laser Ther* **10**: 24–33.
51. Drosner M, Adatto M. (2005) Photo-epilation: guidelines for care from the European Society for Laser Dermatology (ESLD). *J Cosmet Laser Ther* **7**: 33–38.
52. Fournier N. (2008) Hair removal on dark-skinned patients with pneumatic skin flattening (PSF) and a high-energy Nd:YAG laser. *J Cosmet Laser Ther* **10**: 210–212.
53. Narukar VA. (2005) Photopneumatic pixilation: demonstration of a novel approach to light based hair reduction. *Lasers Surg Med* **S17**: 245.
54. Kilmer SL. (2005) Validation of a radically new technology for permanent hair reduction. *Lasers Surg Med* **S17**: 284.
55. Hamzavi I, Tan E, Shapiro J, *et al.* (2007) A randomized bilateral vehicle controlled study of eflornithine cream combined with laser treatment versus laser treatment alone for facial hirsutism in women. *J Am Acad Dermatol* **57**: 54–59.
56. Town G, Ash C. (2009) Measurement of home-use laser and intense pulsed light systems for hair removal: preliminary report. *J Cosmet Laser Ther* **11**: 157–168.

Chapter 8

Ablative Laser Resurfacing in the Asian Skin

Chee-Leok Goh*

Introduction

Wrinkles, dyschromia and telangiectasias are unwanted features of photoaging. Actinic keratoses and skin cancers may also result from photodamage. Scarring from severe acne, surgery, or trauma often becomes accentuated with aging. These skin changes cause disfigurement, often affecting the quality of life, and prompt patients to seek advice about treatment. However, wrinkles, actinic keratoses, and photodamaged changes are less common in the Asian skin. Acne scarring is the main reason most Asian patients seek skin resurfacing treatments.

Skin rejuvenation treatments include topical retinoids, bleaching agents, chemical peeling, fractional photothermolysis, ablative laser resurfacing, and dermabrasion. In addition, some scars and wrinkles can be corrected by excision, subcision, and dermal fillers. These treatments are often used in combination to obtain optimal outcomes.

The newer lasers, including the fractional photothermolysis devices, are now preferred in the treatment of wrinkles and scars and in skin rejuvenation, because when compared to ablative laser resurfacing they cause less morbidity and less severe side effects, especially in the darker skin phototypes. However, their efficaciousness is inferior to the conventional ablative laser resurfacing devices, e.g. the carbon dioxide (CO_2) and the erbium:YAG (Er:YAG) lasers.

*Senior Consultant Dermatologist, National Skin Centre, Singapore.

Clinical Professor, National University of Singapore. Adjunct Professor, Duke-NUS Graduate Medical School.

Indications for Ablative Laser Resurfacing

Ablative laser resurfacing retains a useful role in treating severe wrinkles and atrophic scars that have not responded adequately to other treatment modalities, including nonablative lasers and fractional photothermolysis. It remains the most effective treatment for photodamage, intrinsic wrinkling, acne scars, chickenpox scars, and traumatic scars. The CO_2 laser at 10,600 nm is recognized as an effective method for skin resurfacing for wrinkles and scars. It is efficient and provides good control of bleeding during the resurfacing procedure.

In Asian countries, ablative lasers are predominantly used for the treatment of post-acne scars rather than wrinkles.[1] This is in contrast to Western countries, where ablative resurfacing is predominantly used for wrinkles.

In our patients, CO_2 laser resurfacing provides mild to moderate improvement for acne scars and better outcomes for rhytides. In a study from Singapore, all patients noticed some improvement in their scars and rhytides postoperatively. At six months postoperatively, 25% of the patients achieved minimal improvement (<25% clearance) of their acne scars and 37% had moderate improvement (25–50% clearance). At 12 months, 83% of the patients had moderate improvement (25–50% clearance) and 17% had good improvement. It appears that patients with acne scars continued to show improvement over the 12-month period.[1]

The introduction of scanners has allowed resurfacing of large skin areas. Traditional ablative laser resurfacing offers reliable, predictable outcomes compared with nonablative lasers, which may offer some benefit, but whose potential may have been exaggerated.

Disadvantages of Ablative Laser Resurfacing

These are the long downtime and the requirement of long leave to recover from the laser procedure. About two weeks is needed for re-epithelialization (Fig. 8.1). Postoperative erythema occurs in all patients and lasts for 3–6 months; other side effects include post-inflammatory hyperpigmentation (up to 30–50% of patients, more often in Asian skin) and persistent hypopigmentation (occurring in 5–10% and tends to occur 10–12 mth post ablation). In addition, scarring may occur if the operator is overzealous in the resurfacing procedure. Other complications include secondary bacterial infection and recrudescence of herpes simplex infection.

Erythema is a common postoperative complication.[1] All our patients in the initial six weeks post treatment experienced erythema, but this cleared completely over six months after laser resurfacing. Hyperpigmentation has been reported to occur in 5–50% of patients after CO_2 laser resurfacing and is mainly related to patient skin type, especially among the darker-skinned patients postoperatively. About 25% of our patients experienced post-inflammatory hyperpigmentation (PIH) from six weeks postoperatively, with about 15% having moderately severe hyperpigmentation (Fig. 8.2). From our study, it appears that post-inflammatory hyperpigmentation following laser resurfacing in our Asian patients may not be as frequent as expected, but this pigmentation may be severe in those affected. The pigmentation tends to clear slowly over the next 6–12 months. Patients should be warned of the potential of moderate post-inflammatory hyperpigmentation following laser resurfacing. Vigilant sun protection, use of a broad-spectrum sunscreen and bleaching agents, e.g. hydroquinone cream, may help to reduce the severity and frequency of PIH.

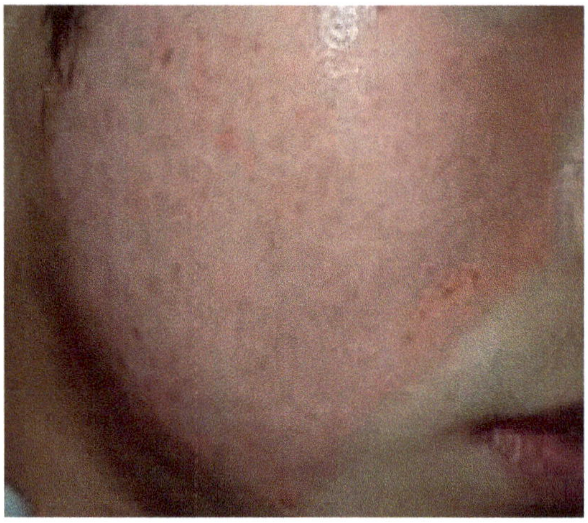

Figure 8.1.

Immidate skin reaction following ablative CO_2 laser resurfacing. The skin is raw and red and the downtime is about 2 weeks post laser treatment.

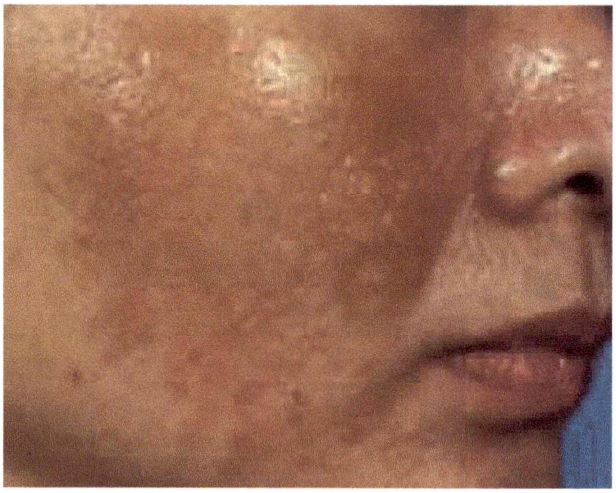

Figure 8.2.

Post-inflammatory hyperpigmentation occuring 3 months after ablative CO_2 laser resurfacing. A common complication observed in dark skin types.

Mechanism of Action of Ablative Laser Resurfacing

The traditional high energy pulsed or scanned CO_2 (10,600 nm) and the Er:YAG (2940 nm) lasers provide precise skin vaporization and predictable outcomes.[2] The superpulsed lasers have high pulse energies to maximize tissue vaporization, as well as a pulse duration of less than 1 millisecond (ms), which is less than the thermal relaxation time of the skin, following the principles of selective photothermolysis.[3]

The ability to control the epidermal vaporization depth with minimal damage to the papillary dermis is a prerequisite for successful, char-free, facial skin resurfacing. In the past, multiple ablative passes were recommended where moderately severe thermal damage was inflicted on the dermis. This resulted in severe morbidity and complications. The later ablative lasers were able to confine ablation to a thin layer (20–50 microns, μ) and deliver enough energy to vaporize tissue in a time shorter than the thermal relaxation time of the skin (1 ms), e.g. the Ultrapulse™ and the Silk-Touch™ (flash-scanners) coupled to a CO_2 laser. The Silk-Touch™ has an opticomechanical flash-scanner and the laser tube is pumped electronically to produce high-power, repetitive, short pulses. The special scanner focuses and scans the laser beam in a spiral pattern for short exposure dwell times of < 1 ms.

Histopathologic studies have shown that the depths of ablation are 20–30μ and 30–50μ after one pass using pulsed and scanning laser technology respectively; the residual thermal damage was 20–40μ per pass, but did not increase to more than 150μ on the third pass.[4] The residual thermal damage produced by the newer CO_2 laser technology is controlled by the pulse duration and produces controlled heating of the dermis.[5] Controlled dermal heating is very important for good clinical results in the treatment of photodamaged skin.

The degree of residual thermal damage (not the depth of tissue ablation) following laser resurfacing is very important for long-lasting clinical improvement. The thermal effect accounts for visible collagen shrinkage and immediate tightening of the skin

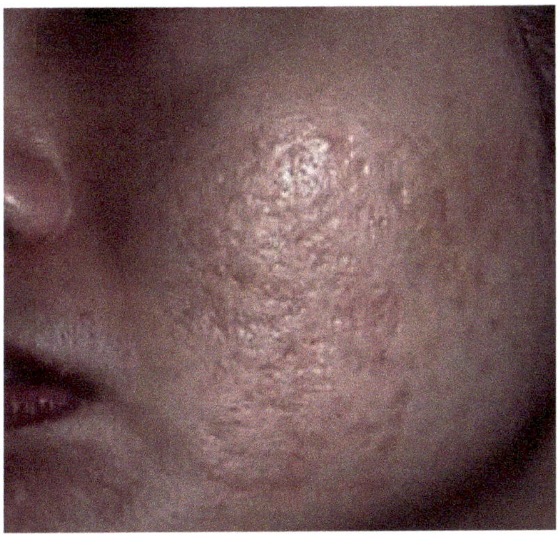

(a)

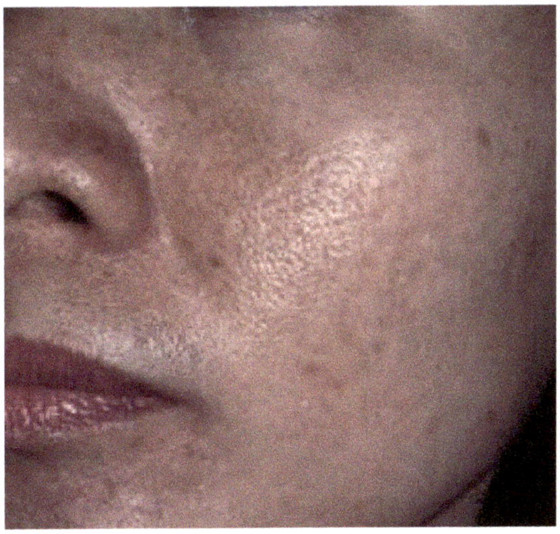

(b)

Figure 8.3.

(a) Atrophic acne scars on cheeks. (b) 1 year post-ablative CO_2 laser resurfacing using the Silk-Touch™, Sharplan laser: 200 mm handpiece, 8 mm spot size, 18 watts, on time: 0.53 sec, off time: 0.40 sec, single pass showing significant improvement.

(Fig. 8.3). CO_2 laser treatment leads to the formation of granulation tissue at day 30 and new collagen formation (fibroplasia) at day 100 post treatment, which seems to be dependent on the depth of the zone of thermal damage.[5]

Ablative Laser Resurfacing Treatment Outcomes

The most common indication for ablative laser resurfacing in Asian patients is the improvement of post-acne scars. The treatment outcome for scars is generally less effective than for wrinkles. Improvement ranges from 30–50% for scars, whereas better results of up to 70% can be achieved with some wrinkles.

CO_2 laser surgery seems to give good results for all scar types, but is better for saucer-shaped distensible areas, rather than pitted scars. Atrophic facial scars,[6] hypertrophic, and traumatic scars can also be ablated with significant improvement of their appearance by blending the texture and color. Perioral and peri-orbital rhytides respond best to treatment, whereas the nasolabial folds do not seem to improve significantly.[6]

Patient Selection and Technique

It is important to carry out a detailed assessment in the initial consultation to select patients who are likely to respond to treatment and to minimize complications. The patient's skin type is important as complications from skin pigmentation are more likely to occur in dark skin types. Stringent sun avoidance and use of sunscreen and prophylactic topical bleaching agents may be useful.

Other important points to note include previous therapies (e.g. oral retinoids, chemical peels, dermabrasion, laser resurfacing, and any previous reactive or permanent post-treatment side effects, for instance, pig mentation problems, keloids, etc.).

Preoperative counseling also ensures that expectations are reasonable and possible risks understood.

Anesthesia is always required for ablative laser resurfacing. For superficial resurfacing, topical anesthesia, e.g. EMLA® cream, a eutectic mixture of 2.5% lidocaine and 2.5% prilocaine, may suffice. However, regional nerve blocks are necessary for deeper ablation and when resurfacing a large area.

The Asian skin has a high propensity to develop post-inflammatory hyperpigmentation. Hence deep ablative dermal resurfacing should be avoided. One to two passes (depending on the fluence used), achieving not more than 120 μ skin ablation, should suffice. One can repeat the resurfacing procedure one year later if the need arises.

During the procedure, ablated skin may be rubbed off to improve epithelialization. However, other authorities prefer to leave the ablated skin as a dressing. There is no evidence-based study to suggest which is better.

Preoperative Care

A study has shown that there is no need for the use of hydroquinone, retinoic acid, or glycolic acid before treatment.[7] Hydroquinone penetration to reach the deep follicular melanocytes, which are responsible for postoperative hyperpigmentation, is questionable. Clinical experience, however, suggests that pre-treatment is important in darker skin types, and topical hydroquinone is often prescribed pre- and postoperatively to reduce PIH. The usual pre-treatment regimen includes hydroquinone, tretinoin cream, or alpha-hydroxy acids and a broad-spectrum sunscreen during the day.

It is standard practice that all ablative laser resurfacing patients need to be started on oral antiviral therapy, e.g. acyclovir, two days prior to the procedure and continuing for 10–14 days until complete re-epithelialization, regardless of the previous history of herpes simplex. The majority of infectious complications associated with this procedure are related to herpetic outbreaks.

The use of prophylactic oral antimicrobials is optional, but with the increasing risk of infections, some dermatologists routinely prescribe prophylactic oral antibiotics, e.g. cephalexin. Patients are also started on an antibiotic one day prior to the procedure for a total of five days.

Faster healing has been shown in patients given antifungals (e.g. fluconazole) to cover the overgrowth of yeast (one dose on the day after the procedure and another dose after one week).

Postoperative Care

Post-treatment swelling and soreness may persist for 10–14 days. Treated areas usually heal in approximately one week, and the post-treatment inflammation resolves over the following six weeks, but can take up to six months. Erythema may take months to resolve, depending on the depth of resurfacing. The deeper the tissue injury, the more persistent the erythema.

Postoperative wound care consists of semi-occlusive dressings ("closed" technique) or petrolatum-based ointment ("open" technique) until full skin re-epithelialization. The "closed" technique may be advantageous over the "open" technique because of faster re-epithelialization and less pain and burning.[8] On the other hand, the majority of infections occur in the setting of occlusive dressings and develop within the first 10 days of laser treatment. Therefore, a semi-closed technique, combining the advantages of both open and closed techniques, is often adopted, whereby the wound is occluded for 48–72 hours and, after that time, an open technique of applying moisturizing creams is instituted.

A topical antimicrobial is best avoided as it may produce local irritation. This may prolong the recovery time and increase the risk of adverse effects, such as erythema and hyperpigmentation.

In order to minimize postoperative hyperpigmentation, a bleaching preparation with 2–4% hydroquinone or combination regimens (containing hydroquinone, fluocinolone acetonide, and tretinoin) may be prescribed after full reepithelialization has occurred. The patient is also advised to avoid excessive sun exposure and to use sunscreen regularly.

Complications of Ablative CO_2 Laser Resurfacing

The incidence of long-lasting complications is low when the ablative devices are used in experienced hands. However, even with optimal laser settings and appropriate use of occlusive dressings to facilitate wound healing, complications can occur. Complications can be minimized with patient education and early recognition and management.[9–12]

Complications can be divided into short- and long-term problems. Short term complications include transient erythema, pruritus, milia, acneiform eruptions, infections, e.g. herpes simplex, bacterial or yeast infections, and post-inflammatory hyperpigmentation. Long-term complications include hypopigmentation and permanent scarring. Hypopigmentation may worsen with time and is a late complication that most commonly appears following aggressive resurfacing in areas with thin skin such as the neck. It is related to the depth of tissue injury during the procedure. Pigment loss is permanent and may be due to injury to the deep follicular melanocytes.

The injudicious use of moisturizers may lead to acne and milia formation. Infections with herpes simplex virus can be treated with acyclovir or valaciclovir. Gram-positive and negative infections usually appear at day 7 postoperatively, and can be treated with oral antibiotics, e.g. ciprofloxacin.

Erbium:Yag Laser Resurfacing

The pulsed Er:YAG laser with the unique feature of maximal water absorption (water absorption coefficient is 16 times greater than the CO_2 laser), and therefore with minimal optical penetration depth and thermal damage, has proven to be efficacious in the treatment of mild to moderate superficial rhytides and scars.[13,14] The Er:YAG laser penetrates to a depth of 5 μ/pass with an energy fluence of 2.8 J/cm^2.[15,16] This infrared spectrum (2940 nm) provides very precise ablation, because of its high selectivity of tissue water and negligible thermal damage. In contrast, with CO_2 lasers a more significant coagulation necrosis occurs (20–40 *μ*/pass). The characteristics of a wavelength with maximal water absorption, a short time duration (< 1 ms), and sufficient fluence place the Er:YAG laser as the optimum ablative device for fine and superficial resurfacing of the skin. Pinpoint bleeding appears after 4–5 passes (depending on the spot size and energy fluence), with exposure of the dermo-epidermal junction, and the laser treatment is usually stopped. Therefore, bleeding is a problem in the treatment of deeper wrinkles with the Er:YAG laser and forces the end of treatment at a more superficial depth, thus preventing the complications seen with CO_2 lasers.

The main advantages of the Er:YAG over the CO_2 laser are reduced thermal damage, shorter recovery time, less postoperative erythema, and less anesthesia requirement. The reduced thermal damage using the Er:YAG laser means a more precise tissue ablation, but also less profound clinical and histologic improvement in photodamaged skin.

In a bilateral comparison study of 20 patients using the CO_2 and Er:YAG lasers in the treatment of facial rhytides, there were no significant differences in postoperative erythema, pain, or healing time when equal depths of tissue coagulation and ablation were achieved with each type of laser.[16] However, this study showed that while postoperative morbidity was similar, the Er:YAG laser showed less efficacy in general. Fine lines responded very well to this laser, whereas deeper rhytides showed a greater response to CO_2 laser resurfacing.

The Er:YAG laser may improve photodamaged skin in areas off limits to CO_2 laser resurfacing, such as the neck, hands, and chest.[17] It should be noted that darker skin types (especially skin type V), which cannot be treated safely with the CO_2 laser, may be treated more safely with the Er:YAG laser. Patients with chicken pox scars have shown improvement by 55% and those with acne scars by 40% after the use of the pulsed Er:YAG laser.[13]

The treatment technique is similar to that of the CO_2 laser, but the clinical endpoint is bleeding, which alerts one to the fact that the papillary dermis has been reached.

Complications of Erbium:Yag Laser Resurfacing

In general, the Er:YAG laser causes less morbidity than the CO_2 laser, with less postoperative erythema, which usually lasts for 2–4 weeks. Post-inflammatory hyperpigmentation is transient. Late complications, such as hypopigmentation, are seen in fewer patients (4%) when treated with the Er:YAG laser compared to the CO_2 laser.[18] The presence of bleeding forces the surgeon to discontinue laser treatment and therefore prevents serious complications.

Long-Pulsed Erbium:Yag Laser

Less adverse sequelae are seen with the use of erbium:YAG lasers but the degree of improvement that can be obtained with the CO_2 laser cannot be achieved. Long-pulsed erbium:YAG lasers (LP Er:YAG) have been developed to deliver increased thermal effects to tissue. These lasers can improve clinical outcomes while still allowing for diminished erythema and improved wound healing.[19]

One study reported that clinical improvement was equal for both the ultrapulsed CO_2 ($UPCO_2$) laser and LP Er:YAG laser, with an average improvement in photoaging scores of 53%.[19] There was a tendency toward faster healing and less edema on the LP Er:YAG treated side. Histologic examination of tissue taken after the final erbium pass revealed similar thermal damage for the two lasers, with an average depth of 28.2 μ on the $UPCO_2$-treated side versus 23.8 μ on the LP Er:YAG-treated side. Both showed evidence of new collagen formation three months after the procedure; the average depth of new collagen formation for the $UPCO_2$-treated side was 35 μ and for the LP Er:YAG-treated side was 23 μ.

Conclusion

Ablative laser resurfacing remains the gold standard for laser skin resurfacing for scars and rhytides. The high morbidity rates and long downtime limit its use. Caution is needed in dark skin types as the risk of PIH is high. Hence, fractional laser resurfacing has gained in popularity. There is still a role for ablative laser resurfacing, e.g. when newer technologies do not achieve the expected results. With proper patient selection, conservative treatment protocols and good pre- and postoperative skin care, most complications can be prevented or moderated.

References

1. Goh CL, Khoo L. (2002) Laser skin resurfacing treatment outcome of facial scars and wrinkles in Asians with skin type III/IV with the Unipulse CO_2 laser system. *Singapore Med J* **43**: 28–32.
2. Ross EV, Domankevitz Y, Skrobal M, *et al.* (1996) Effects of CO_2 laser pulse in ablation and thermal damage: implications for skin resurfacing. *Lasers Surg Med* **19**: 123–129.
3. Goldman MP, Fitzpatrick RE. (1994) CO_2 laser surgery. In: Baxter SH (ed.), *Cutaneous Laser Surgery: The Art and Science of Selective Photothermolysis*, St Louis, MO: Mosby-Year Book, pp. 198–258.
4. Kauvar ANB, Geronemus RG. (1997) Histology of laser resurfacing. *Dermatol Clin* **15**: 459–467.
5. Walsh J, Flotte T, Anderson R, *et al.* (1988) Pulsed CO_2 laser tissue ablation: effect of tissue type and pulse duration on thermal damage. *Lasers Surg Med* **8**: 108–118.
6. Alster TS, West TB. (1996) Resurfacing of atrophic facial scars with a high-energy pulsed carbon dioxide laser. *Dermatol Surg* **22**: 151–155.
7. West TB, Alster TS. (1999) Effect of pretreatment on the incidence of hyperpigmentation following cutaneous CO_2 laser resurfacing. *Dermatol Surg* **25**: 15–17.
8. Weinstein S, Ramirez O, Pozner J. (1998) Postoperative care following carbon dioxide laser resurfacing. *Dermatol Surg* **24**: 51–56.
9. Nanni CA, Alster TS. (1998) Complications of cutaneous laser surgery. *Dermatol Surg* **24**: 209–213.
10. Berstein LJ, Kauvar ANB, Grossman M, *et al.* (1997) The short- and long-term side effects of carbon dioxide laser resurfacing. *Dermatol Surg* **23**: 519–525.
11. Nanni CA, Alster TS. (1998) Complications of carbon dioxide laser resurfacing. *Dermatol Surg* **24**: 315–320.
12. Fulton JE. (1998) Complications of laser resurfacing. Methods of prevention and management. *Dermatol Surg* **24**: 91–99.
13. Young CK. (1997) Resurfacing of pitted facial scars with a pulsed Er:YAG laser. *Dermatol Surg* **23**: 880–883.
14. Perez MI, Bank DE, Silvers D. (1998) Skin resurfacing of the face with the Erbium:YAG laser. *Dermatol Surg* **24**: 653–659.
15. Kaufmann R, Hibst R. (1996) Pulsed Erbium:YAG laser ablation in cutaneous surgery. *Lasers Surg Med* **19**: 324–330.
16. Walsh JT, Jr, Deutsch TF. (1989) Er:YAG laser ablation of tissue: measurement of ablation rates. *Lasers Surg Med* **9**: 327–337.
17. Goldberg DJ, Meine JG. (1998) Treatment of photoaged neck skin with the pulsed Erbium:YAG laser. *Dermatol Surg* **24**: 619–622.
18. Wenstein C. (1999) Erbium laser resurfacing: current concepts. *Plast Reconstr Surg* **103**: 602–616.
19. Newman NB, Lord JL, Ash K, *et al.* (2000) Variable pulse Er:YAG laser skin resurfacing of perioral rhytides and side by side comparison with CO_2 laser. *Lasers Surg Med* **26**: 208–214.

Chapter 9

Nonablative Laser Photorejuvenation in the Asian Skin

Por-Ang*

Introduction

The traditional modalities of skin resurfacing for rhytides, scars, and photoaged skin include dermabrasion, chemical peels, and ablative laser resurfacing with carbon dioxide and erbium:YAG lasers. The presumed mechanisms of clinical improvement from these invasive or ablative modalities are: epidermal ablation, collagen remodeling, and dermal contraction.[1–5] However, these procedures are associated with complications such as prolonged healing and erythema, post-inflammatory pigmentary changes, infection, and scarring. In the last decade, dermatologic surgeons have been exploring the possibility of directly stimulating collagen remodeling without epidermal ablation. This would theoretically eliminate the complications and long downtime of the older invasive procedures. This proposed new concept has been termed *nonablative skin rejuvenation* or *subsurface remodeling.* To achieve this, epidermal protection and sufficiently long wavelengths that can penetrate and injure the dermis are requisites. Many lasers and light sources have been utilized and developed for this purpose. This chapter reviews the available data on these devices, their clinical efficacy, histological effects, and side effects.

*Consultant Dermatologist, Dermatology Associates, Paragon Medical Centre, Singapore.

Lasers and Light Sources

A variety of laser and light sources have been studied for nonablative skin rejuvenation. Some of these are pre-existing equipment, e.g. 1064 nm Q-switched Nd:YAG laser, 585–595 nm pulsed dye laser, and intense pulsed light. Some are lasers specifically developed by the laser manufacturers for this purpose, e.g. 1320 nm Nd:YAG laser, 1450 nm diode laser, and 1540 nm erbium-glass laser. The target chromophore is postulated to be dermal water or hemoglobin.

Skin Conditions Amenable to Treatment with Nonablative Lasers
Scars
Wrinkles
Photoaging
Acne vulgaris
Sebaceous hyperplasia
Skin tightening
Striae distensae
Pores

1064 nm Q-switched (QS) Nd:YAG Laser

One of the earliest nonablative rejuvenation studies assessed the 1064 nm QS Nd:YAG laser. In 1997, Goldberg and Whitworth treated 11 patients simultaneously with the QS Nd:YAG laser, the SilkTouch™ CO_2 laser, and Ultrapulse™ CO_2 laser.[6] They reported 81.8% improvement at three months with the QS

Nd:YAG laser, with 27.2% of patients experiencing improvement to a similar degree with the CO_2 lasers. Interestingly, these patients were those who experienced erythema with the QS Nd:YAG laser, leading to the authors' postulation that perhaps erythema is an indicator of adequate dermal injury required for remodeling.

Subsequently, Goldberg and Metzler[7] used the laser in combination with topical carbon suspension as an exogenous chromophore to enable lower fluences to be used, and Goldberg and Silapunt then did clinical and histologic evaluation of the QS Nd:YAG laser.[8,9] In all these studies, 68–97% showed improvement. However, they were hampered by petechiae immediately after treatment.

585–595 nm Pulsed Dye Laser

Studies on the pulsed dye laser were prompted by observations that it can improve striae distensae and hypertrophic scars, which suggested a beneficial effect on dermal collagen and also anecdotal observations of improved rhytides in patients treated for facial vessels. The target chromophore is hemoglobin in dermal vasculature.

Zelickson *et al*'s study was a combination of two independent and separate studies with different methodologies and assessments, making direct comparison difficult.[10] However, the follow-up periods were 12–14 mth, making it one of the longest. The lasers used were the 450 μs pulsed dye lasers commonly used for vascular lesions. The study reported 40–90% subjective improvement in rhytides, mostly maintained at the end of the follow-up period.

Bjerring *et al.* used a pulsed dye laser with a pulse duration of 350 μs.[11] This laser was developed with the purpose of injuring the dermis without damaging the microvasculature and causing purpura. The increase in collagen production in their study was thought to be due to a low grade inflammatory response in the blood vessels, releasing mediators that stimulate fibroblast activity. Both studies used a single treatment; it remains to be seen if multiple treatments with this laser will lead to better clinical improvement.

Tay *et al.* treated 10 patients with facial wrinkles with the long pulsed dye laser (595 nm, 10 mm spot size, 10 ms pulse duration, 7 J/cm^2, 40 ms cryogen spray, 40 ms delay, single-pass, 30% overlap) on one side with the other side serving as a control.[12] A total of three treatments were given at 2 monthly intervals. At two months after the last treatment, mild to moderate improvement of rhytides was noted in all patients with the peri-orbital area being more responsive to treatment. No clinical changes were noted in the control areas. Treatment was well tolerated with no adverse effects except for transient mild erythema.

Intense Pulsed Light

Intense pulsed lights are flashlamp devices that emit wavelengths of noncoherent light between 550 and 1100 nm. With higher cutoff filters, the shorter wavelengths are blocked and the emitted longer wavelengths can be utilized for generating nonspecific dermal damage. These devices have been used successfully for treatment of vascular lesions.

Goldberg's earlier 2 studies used a higher cutoff filter of 645 nm whereas Bitter suggested that using a lower filter may be better for improving concurrent epidermal lesions such as telangiectasia and flushing.[13–15]

Goldberg and Samady then compared the intense pulsed light using 590 nm and 755 nm cutoff filters and the 1064 nm QS Nd:YAG laser and concluded that there did not seem to be major differences in the efficacy.[16] However, more side effects such as blistering and erythema (>50%) were noted with the shorter wavelength.

1320 nm Nd:YAG Laser

The 1320 nm Nd:YAG laser was the first laser to be manufactured specifically for nonablative skin rejuvenation. The wavelength was selected for its dermal penetration and its significant scattering coefficient, which allows for a larger volume of dermal damage compared to the laser beam size. The target chromophore is dermal water. The studies included two models.

The New Star™ model was associated with blistering and pitted scarring.[17,18] This was thought to be due to excessive or malfunctioning cryogen effect, and/or the absence of a thermal sensor.

The newer CoolTouch™ model incorporated a thermal sensor that measures the epidermal tem-perature. It is thought that the target peak epidermal temperature achieved with the laser should be between 42 and 48ºC, corresponding to an optimal dermal temperature required for injury and remodeling. Since there is individual variability in the baseline epidermal temperature, the laser fluences used need to be adjusted according to the sensor to achieve the peak target epidermal temperature.

The results with the New Star™ model appeared modest and significant improvement was seen only with severe rhytides. However, the more impressive results with the CoolTouch™ studies were tempered by the small study population ($n = 10$) and the largely subjective evaluation.[19–21]

1540 nm Erbium-glass Laser

The erbium glass laser was developed in view of its dermal penetration and its minimal melanin absorption. The two studies reviewed lasers with different pulse emission modes.

Ross *et al.* reported hardly any clinical effect and the biopsies showed dermal fibroplasia in the deep dermis only, which does not correspond to the zone of photodamage.[22] Fournier *et al.* reported subjective and objective improvement with histological evidence of superficial dermal collagen production using their laser system.[23]

1450 nm Diode Laser

The 1450 nm diode laser (Smoothbeam™) was developed for nonablative laser rejuvenation. In addition to its effects on rhytides[24] and scars,[25,26] it was also shown to improve acne[27,28] and sebaceous hyperplasia.[29] In an Asian study using the 1450 nm diode laser for atrophic acne scars, a mean improvement of 15–20% was achieved after 4–6 treatments in 60% of patients[26] (Figs. 9.1 and 9.2). The most common

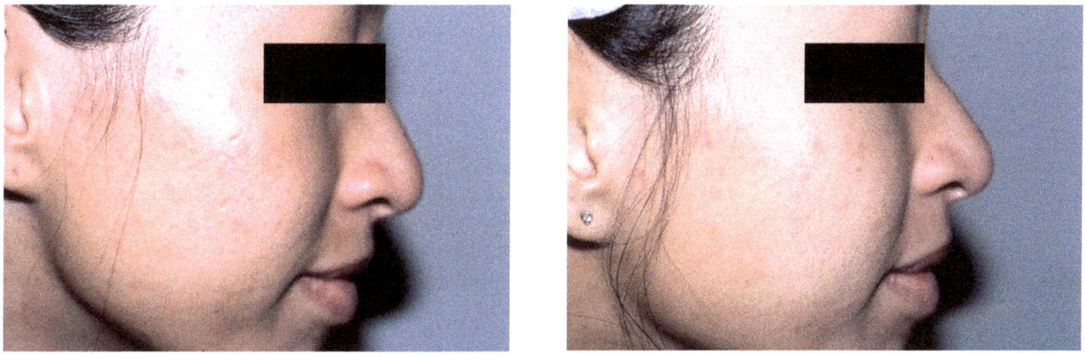

Pre-treatment.
(Courtesy of National Skin Centre.)

1 mth after 2 treatments at monthly intervals.

Figure 9.1.

Smoothbeam™ (1450 nm diode laser) 6 mm spot size, 11 J/cm^2, 40 ms cryogen spray cooling.

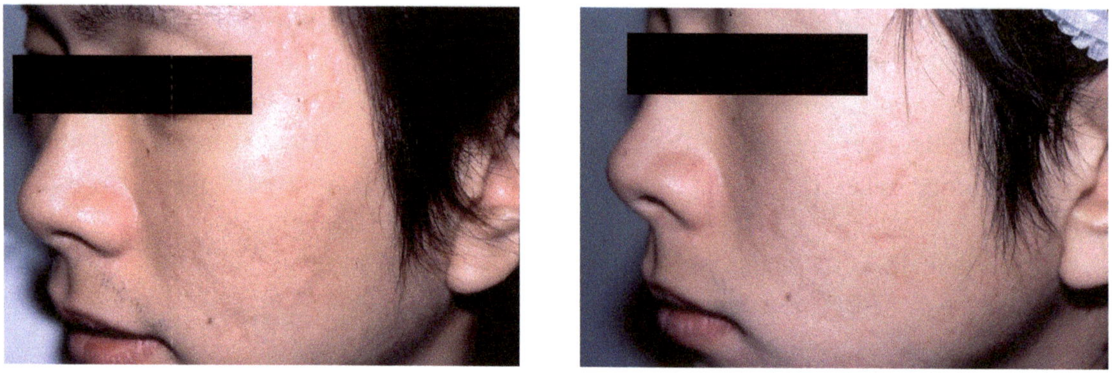

Pre-treatment.
(Courtesy of National Skin Centre.)

1 mth after 3 treatments at monthly intervals.

Figure 9.2.

Smoothbeam™ (1450 nm diode laser) 6 mm spot size, 12 J/cm^2, 40 ms cryogen spray cooling.

side effect in this study was post-inflammatory hyperpigmentation (39%), which appeared to be due to the cryogen spray of the laser.

Long Pulsed Nd:YAG 1064 nm

Some long pulsed Nd:YAG laser systems that are used for hair removal and veins can be used for nonablative laser rejuvenation. Improvements in skin tightening,[30] pores[31] and stretch marks[32] have been noted. Histological evidence of new collagen formation has been reported after the use of this laser.[33]

Anesthesia and Postoperative Care

A topical anesthetic cream, e.g. EMLA,® an eutectic mixture of lidocaine 2.5% and prilocaine 2.5%, is applied an hour before the laser procedure. Eyes are protected with eye shields.

Most patients have mild transient erythema and swelling after nonablative procedures. Because there is no epidermal ablation, the postoperative care is simple and there is usually no need for any aftercare. A mild topical steroid or aloe vera gel for a few days will usually suffice in cases of erythema and swelling.

Side Effects and Complications with Emphasis on the Asian Skin

The risk of side effects with nonablative laser photorejuvenation is low since there is no epidermal ablation. In Asian skin, the risks are post-inflammatory hyperpigmentation (PIH), especially if there are concomitant pigmentary disorders like melasma. PIH may be caused by the heat generated or excessive cryogen spray of certain lasers. Blistering is rare but possible if the fluence used is too high.

Conclusion

Nonablative skin rejuvenation is an attractive concept with the theoretical possibility of stimulating collagen synthesis and remodeling without the complications of traditional skin resurfacing procedures. However, the studies thus far have shown modest and mostly subjective clinical improvement. At present, it is not considered as effective as ablative resurfacing but it does present a viable option for patients who are unwilling to undergo the long downtime or risk the side effects of ablative procedures, and who are prepared to accept multiple treatment sessions and mild improvement. It may also be a useful adjunct to other cosmetic treatments like chemical peels, fillers, and botulinum toxin injection, or as maintenance after ablative therapy.

More recently, the concept of fractional laser resurfacing has been developed, providing faster and more visible clinical improvement, but also with more downtime and side effects compared to the nonablative lasers, although not to the extent of those from ablative laser resurfacing. While it may seem that fractional laser resurfacing may supersede the nonablative procedures, the latter probably will continue to play a role in skin rejuvenation, especially for patients who require minimal risks and downtime.

References

1. Fitzpatrick R, Goldman M, Satur N, *et al.* (1996) Pulsed carbon dioxide laser resurfacing of photoaged skin. *Arch Dermatol* **132**: 395–402.
2. Nelson B, Fader D, Gillard M, *et al.* (1995) Pilot histologic and ultrastructural study of the effects of medium depth chemical facial peels on dermal collagen in patients with actinically damaged skin. *J Am Acad Dermatol* **32**: 472–478.
3. Nelson B, Majmudar G, Griffiths C, *et al.* (1994) Clinical improvement following dermabrasion of photoaged skin correlates with synthesis of collagen I. *Arch Dermatol* **130**: 1136–1140.
4. Green H, Burd E, Nishioka N, *et al.* (1992) Middermal wound healing: a comparison between dermatomal excision and pulsed carbon dioxide laser ablation. *Arch Dermatol* **128**: 639–645.
5. Cotton J, Hood A, Gonin R, *et al.* (1996) Histologic evaluation of preauricular and postauricular human skin after high energy, short-pulse carbon dioxide laser. *Arch Dermatol* **132**: 425–428.
6. Goldberg DJ, Whitworth J. (1997) Laser skin resurfacing with the Q-switched Nd:YAG laser. *Dermatol Surg* **23**: 903–907.
7. Goldberg DJ, Metzler C. (1999) Skin resurfacing utilizing a low fluence Nd:YAG laser. *J Cut Laser Ther* **1**: 23–27.
8. Goldberg DJ, Silapunt S. (2000) Q-switched Nd:YAG laser: rhytid improvement by nonablative dermal remodeling. *J Cut Laser Ther* **2**: 157–160.
9. Goldberg DJ, Silapunt S. (2000) Histologic evaluation of a Q-switched Nd:YAG laser in the nonablative treatment of wrinkles. *Dermatol Surg* **27**: 744–746.
10. Zelickson BD, Kilmer SL, Bernstein E, *et al.* (1999) Pulsed dye laser therapy for sun damaged skin. *Lasers Surg Med* **25**: 229–236.
11. Bjerring P, Clement M, Heickendorff L, *et al.* (2000) Selective nonablative wrinkle reduction by laser. *J Cut Laser Ther* **2**: 9–15.
12. Tay YK, Khoo BP, Tan E, *et al.* (2004) Long pulsed dye laser treatment of facial wrinkles. *J Cosmet Laser Ther* **6**: 131–135.
13. Goldberg DJ, Cutler KB. (2000) Nonablative treatment of rhytids with intense pulsed light. *Lasers Surg Med* **26**: 196–200.
14. Goldberg DJ. (2000) New collagen formation after dermal remodeling with an intense pulsed light source. *J Cut Laser Ther* **2**: 59–61.
15. Bitter PH. (2000) Noninvasive rejuvenation of photodamaged skin using serial full face intense pulsed light treatments. *Dermatol Surg* **26**: 835–843.
16. Goldberg DJ, Samady JA. (2001) Intense pulsed light and Nd:YAG laser nonablative treatment of facial rhytids. *Lasers Surg Med* **28**: 141–144.
17. Menaker GM, Wrone DA, Williams RM, *et al.* (1999) Treatment of facial rhytids with a nonablative laser: a clinical and histologic study. *Dermatol Surg* **25**: 440–444.
18. Kelly KM, Nelson JS, Lask G, *et al.* (1999) Cryogen spray cooling in combination with nonablative laser treatment of facial rhytides. *Arch Dermatol* **135**: 691–694.
19. Goldberg DJ. (1999) Non ablative subsurface remodelling: a clinical and histologic evaluation of 1320 nm Nd:YAG laser. *J Cut Laser Ther* **1**: 153–157.
20. Goldberg DJ. (2000) Full face nonablative dermal remodelling with a 1320 nm Nd:YAG laser. *Dermatol Surg* **26**: 915–918.
21. Trelles MS, Allones I, Luna R. (2001) Facial rejuvenation with a nonablative 1320 nm Nd:YAG laser: a preliminary clinical and histologic evaluation. *Dermatol Surg* **27**: 111–116.
22. Ross EV, Sajben FP, Hsia J, *et al.* (2001) Nonablative skin remodelling: selective dermal heating with a mid-infrared laser and contact cooling combination. *Lasers Surg Med* **26**: 186–195.
23. Fournier N, Dahan S, Barneon G, *et al.* (2001) Nonablative remodelling: clinical, histologic, ultrasound imaging and profilometric evaluation of a 1540 nm Er:glass laser. *Dermatol Surg* **27**: 799–806.

24. Tanzi EL, Williams CM, Alster TS. (2003) Treatment of facial rhytides with a nonablative 1450 nm diode laser: a controlled clinical and histologic study. *Dermatol Surg* **29**: 124–128.
25. Tanzi EL, Alster TS. (2004) Comparison of a 1450 nm diode laser and a 1320 nm Nd:YAG laser in the treatment of atrophic facial scars: a prospective clinical and histologic study. *Dermatol Surg* **30**: 152–157.
26. Chua SH, Ang P, Khoo LSW, *et al.* (2004) Nonablative 1450 nm diode laser in the treatment of facial atrophic acne scars in type IV to V Asian skin: a prospective clinical study. *Dermatol Surg* **30**: 1287–1291.
27. Bernstein E. (2009) Double-pass, low-fluence laser treatment using a large spot-size 1450 nm laser improves acne. *Lasers Surg Med* **41**: 116–121.
28. Noborio R, Niishida E, Morita A. (2009) Clinical effect of low-energy double pass 1450 nm laser treatment for acne in Asians. *Photodermatol Photoimmunol Photomed* **25**: 3–7.
29. No D, MCClaren, Chotzen V, *et al.* (2004) Sebaceous hyperplasia treated with a 1450 nm diode laser. *Dermatol Surg* **30**: 382–384.
30. Key D. (2007) Single-treatment skin tightening by radiofrequency and long-pulsed 1064 nm Nd:YAG laser compared. *Lasers Surg Med* **39**: 169–175.
31. Lee CN, Kim YJ, Lee HS, *et al.* (2009) Effects of Q-switched and long-pulsed 1064 nm Nd:YAG laser on enlarged facial pores. *Photodermatol Photoimmunol Photomed* **25**: 328–330.
32. Goldman A, Rossato F, Prati C. (2008) Stretch marks: treatment using the 1064 nm Nd:YAG laser. *Dermatol Surg* **34**: 686–692.
33. Dayan S, Damrose JF, Bhattacharyya TK, *et al.* (2003) Histological evaluations following 1064 nm Nd:YAG laser resurfacing. *Lasers Surg Med* **33**: 126–131.

Chapter 10

Fractionated Lasers in the Asian Skin

Sze-Hon Chua*

Introduction

Until recently, there have been two categories of laser skin rejuvenation — conventional ablative and nonablative. Conventional ablative laser resurfacing destroys confluent areas of the skin and gives good results, but is associated with prolonged downtime due to the resultant open wound. Side effects are significant and include a high incidence of post-inflammatory hyperpigmentation (PIH) and delayed hypopigmentation, especially in the darker skin phototypes, that is often permanent. Nonablative laser rejuvenation, on the other hand, does not damage the epidermis and therefore poses minimal risk, but at best produces only marginal clinical improvement.

Fractional photothermolysis (FP), a new concept of how laser energy may be delivered to the skin, was first introduced in 2004 by Manstein and colleagues using a prototype nonablative device.[1] The machine emits laser light in a fractional manner to cause microscopic zones of injury, termed by the authors microthermal zones (MTZ) (Fig. 10.1). This first study, which evaluated the use of FP in the treatment of photoaged forearm skin and peri-orbital rhytides, found the novel approach to be clinically effective. The effectiveness of the fractional approach to lasering was subsequently validated by many other authors with expanding clinical indications for situations where FP may be effective.

*Senior Consultant, Chief, Dermatological Surgery and Laser Unit, National Skin Centre, Singapore.

Concept Behind Fractional Photothermolysis

The scientific concept behind FP involves delivering laser energy to the skin via microbeams rather than macrobeams. The microbeams generally have diameters of less than 300 microns. The pixelated laser light induces thermal injury to the epidermis and underlying dermis in strictly confined microscopic columns or zones, rather than in the broad macroscopic and confluent zones that are characteristic of conventional ablative and nonablative laser resurfacing. Creating microscopic, coagulated columns of tissue deep in the dermis with surrounding healthy tissues eliminates the need for patients to deal with a raw surface wound and its associated prolonged recovery time.

Subsequent wound healing repairs the damaged epidermis and dermis, while the spared, viable, normal tissue surrounding the thermally damaged zones accelerates the wound-healing process by initiating basal epidermal stem cell activity and rapid re-epithelialization. The columns of injury may also serve as channels for the transepidermal elimination of epidermal melanin, damaged keratinocytes, and other dermal debris. Dermal-epidermal signaling continues to promote dermal remodeling and new collagen formation for several months after treatment.

The choice of wavelength is deliberate and targets water as a chromophore rather than hemoglobin or melanin. Choosing such wavelengths allow for areas of thermal injury to be confined to a multitude of water-rich targets such as epidermal keratinocytes,

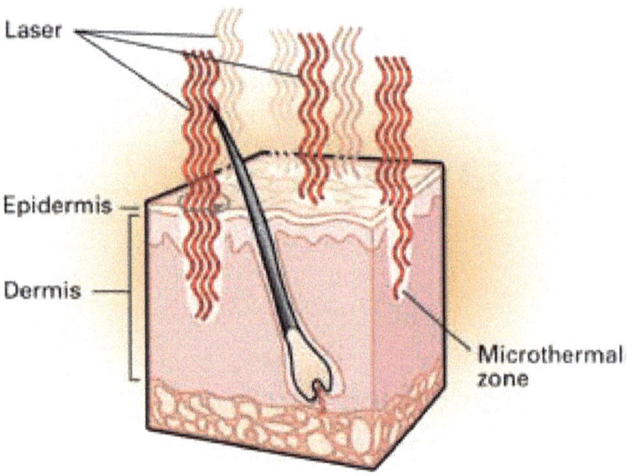

Figure 10.1.

Fractional photothermolysis is a novel concept of delivering laser energy to the skin via microbeams to induce thermal injury to the epidermis and underlying dermis in strictly confined microscopic zones rather than in broad macroscopic and confluent zones.

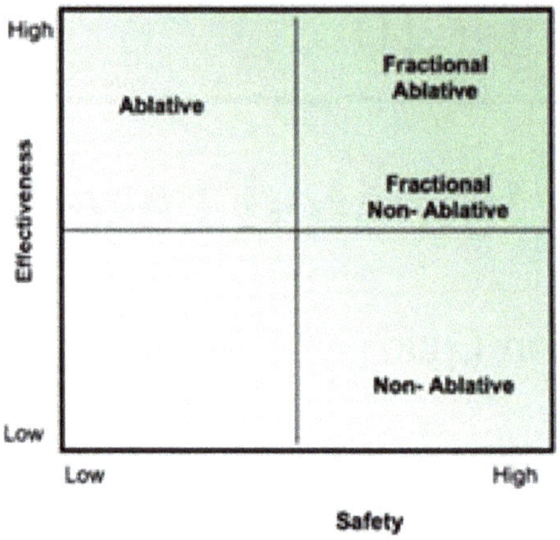

Figure 10.2.

Comparative safety and efficacy of skin rejuvenation technologies.

collagen, and blood vessels located at varying depths throughout the skin.

The concept of FP was initially applied to nonablative wavelengths in the mid-infrared spectrum, e.g. 1550 nm (erbium-doped fiber laser) and 1540 nm (erbium-glass laser). Subsequently, FP was successfully applied to ablative wavelengths such as 10,600 nm (CO_2 laser) and 2940 nm (Er:YAG laser).

Currently available commercial examples of nonablative fractional lasers include Fraxel Re:store™ — Reliant (1550 nm), Lux1540 Fractional™ — Palomar (1540 nm), and Mosaic™ — Lutronic (1540 nm). Currently available commercial examples of ablative fractional lasers include Mixto SX™ — Lasering (10,600 nm), DeepFX™ — Lumenis (10,600 nm), Fraxel Re:pair™ — Reliant (10,600 nm), Juvia™ — Ellipse (10,600 nm), SmartXide DOT™ — Eclipsemed (10,600 nm), Pixel 2940™ — Alma (2940 nm), and ProFractional™ — Sciton (2940 nm).

Theoretically, clinical benefits from FP should mirror those of conventional resurfacing, albeit in a more gradual and staged manner requiring multiple treatments as a trade-off for quicker recovery and fewer complications, especially dyspigmentation. Clinical improvements are expected in the areas of epidermal dyschromias from epidermal renewal and skin texture improvement, and in rhytides and atrophic acne scars from the formation of new collagen in the dermis. The relative safety and efficacy of FP compared to traditional resurfacing technologies is illustrated in Fig. 10.2. The gentler nature of FP and the ability to adjust for energy levels and treatment densities also allows for treatment of off-facial sites, which traditionally are at high risk of scarring after conventional ablative laser resurfacing.

Proof of Concept

Rapid Healing Time

Rapid healing time after FP is well proven by numerous clinical studies and validated by histological evaluation.

For nonablative fractional photothermolysis (NAFP), erythema after treatment is typical and lasts for 3–7 days (Fig. 10.3). Mild swelling is expected and may last 1–3 days. Unlike conventional ablative laser resurfacing, no blisters, crusting, or oozing occurs. No open wound is created.[1,2] Patients can typically apply

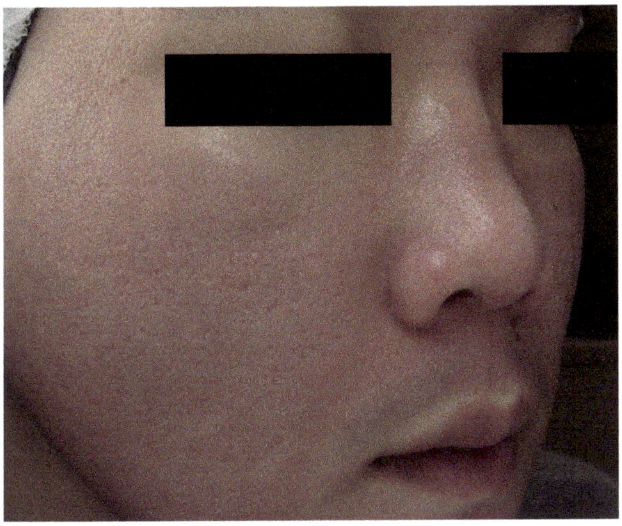

Figure 10.3.

Erythema after nonablative fractional photothermolysis typically lasts 3–7 days.

make-up following treatment and resume normal activities the very next day.

Histologically, epidermal coagulation occurs immediately following NAFP treatment. The stratum corneum remains intact, preserving epidermal barrier function and minimizing the risk of secondary bacterial infection. The dermis is thermally damaged by well-demarcated columns of coagulation (MTZ). By 72 hours, re-epithelialization is complete and the basement membrane is partially restored. Melanin content within the MTZ has been shown to be significantly higher than in surrounding tissue, which is subsequently eliminated together with the damaged keratinocytes and dermal contents transepidermally. By 7 days, the thermally damaged epidermal debris is completely exfoliated and, by three months, the MTZs are replaced by new collagen.[2,3]

For ablative fractional photothermolysis (AFP), erythema is more prolonged and may last 1–4 weeks. Mild swelling over the treated areas is typical and lasts 1–3 days. No blisters, purpura, or bleeding occurs. The pixelated surface wound is rapidly filled with serous exudates forming minute, discrete crusts. Oozing may occur if aggressive parameters are used, causing the epidermis to be more extensively

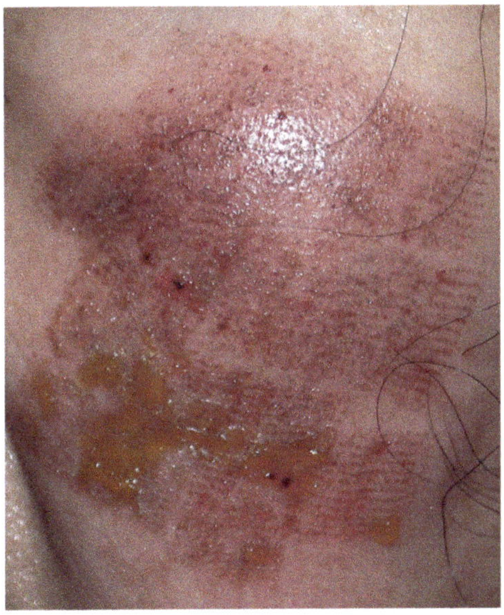

Figure 10.4.

This 52-year-old woman, who was treated with the Mixto SX™ fractional CO_2 laser using more intense treatment parameters (180 micron spot size, 14 watts, index 6, treatment density 20%), developed ooziness and excessive facial swelling on day 2 after treatment.

vaporized and the dermis to be more extensively damaged (Fig. 10.4). The pixelated crusts usually occur after day 2–3 and fall off after 5–7 days.

Clinical Effectiveness

The clinical effectiveness of FP has been shown by many studies. The situations where FP (NAFP and AFP) has been demonstrated to be effective include fine wrinkling and textural changes associated with chronic photoaging[1,4–7] and acne scarring.[8–10]

The clinical improvements have been supported by histological and electron microscopic evidence of new collagen formation.

Safety

The low risk of FP has been verified by numerous studies. Short-term complications may be encountered in 10% of patients.[11] Common complications

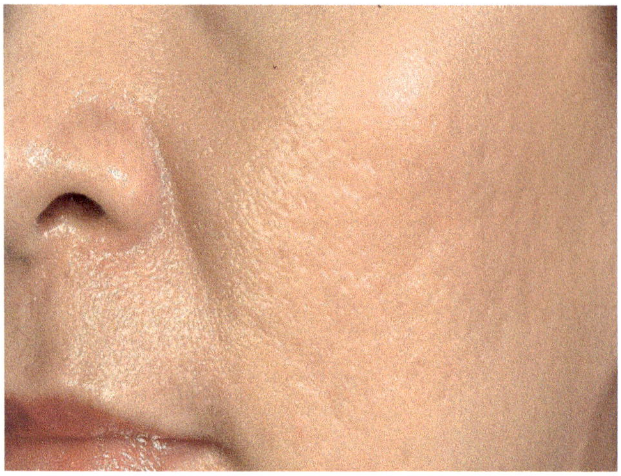

Before treatment.

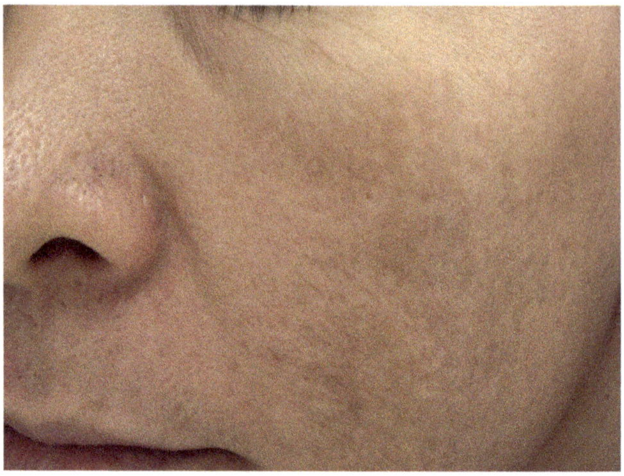

After treatment.

Figure 10.5.

PIH occurs in 5–10% of patients treated with FP and is related to the use of more intense treatment parameters and failure of sun-protection post treatment.

include acneiform eruptions and reactivation of herpes simplex virus (HSV) infection. In Asian skin, post-inflammatory hyperpigmentation occurs in about 5–10% of patients and is related to the use of more intense treatment parameters[12] and failure to practice adequate sun protection post treatment (Fig. 10.5). More serious complications, such as blistering leading to permanent scarring, are rare if recommended treatment protocols and proper lasering techniques are used. Prolonged erythema lasting several weeks is also related to the intensity of the treatment administered.

The safety of FP is extended even to treatment of off-facial sites such as the neck, chest, and hands.[13,14] These areas are at high risk of scarring and hypopigmentation if treated with conventional ablative laser resurfacing.

Clinical Indications

The established clinical indications for FP (both NAFP and AFP) are photoaging[1,4–7] (Fig. 10.6), acne scars[8–10] (Figs. 10.7, 10.8), and surgical scars.[15,16] AFP may be superior to NAFP, although NAFP offers the advantage of less downtime compared with AFP.

Additional indications for NAFP include melasma,[17–19] hypertrophic scars,[20] poikiloderma of Civatte,[21] and colloid milium.[22] While several studies have reported effective treatment of melasma with NAFP, there may be limitations, especially in Asian patients, due to the variability of response rate, higher risk of PIH, and high recurrence rates after treatment.[23] Additional indications for AFP include treatment of skin laxity, as skin tightening occurs after treatment.[24]

Patient Selection

Absolute contraindications include patients who have recently been on systemic isotretinoin therapy in the last six months and patients with active skin infections or open wounds. Relative contraindications include patients who are keloid prone, recent sun exposure/tanning, and patients who still have active acne. Patients with a past history of HSV infections will require antiviral prophylaxis, e.g. with acyclovir,

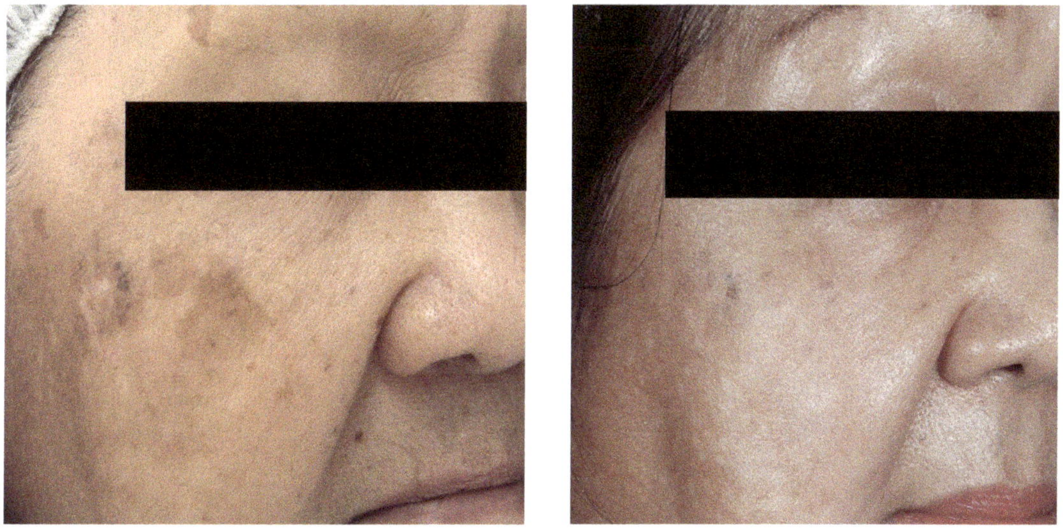

Before treatment. After treatment.

Figure 10.6.

A 72-year-old woman with moderate facial photoaging showing significant improvement in superficial dyschromias, fine wrinkling, and skin texture after 3 sessions with the Mixto SX™ fractional CO_2 laser. Treatment parameters used: 300 micron spot size, power 12–14 watts, index 6, treatment density 20–40%.

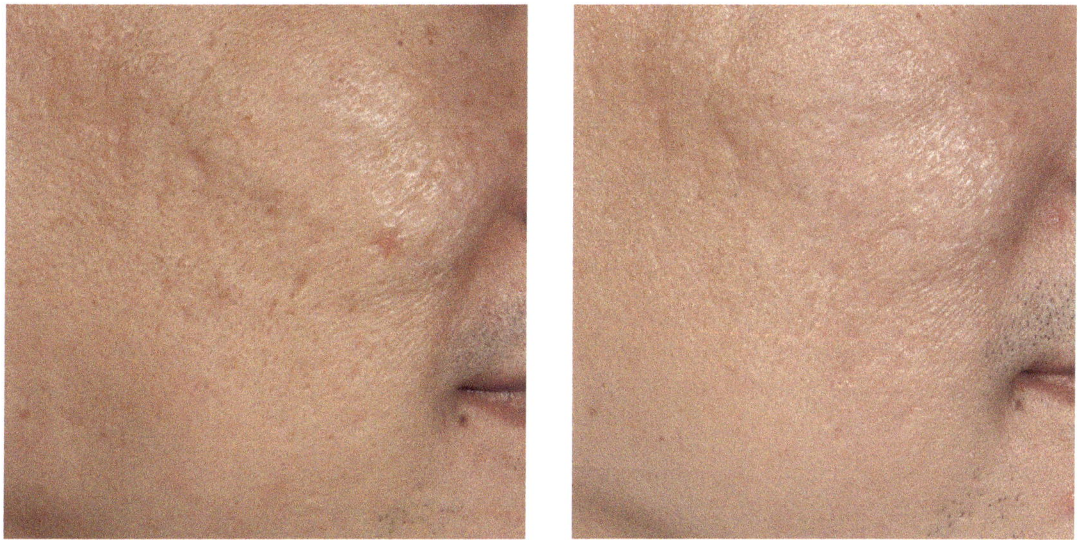

Before treatment. After treatment.

Figure 10.7.

A 45-year-old man with atrophic acne scars showing significant clinical improvement after 4 treatment sessions with the Fraxel:Restore™ (1550 nm erbium-doped fiber) laser. Treatment parameters used: fluence 70 mJ, treatment level 7–10, treatment density 20–30%.

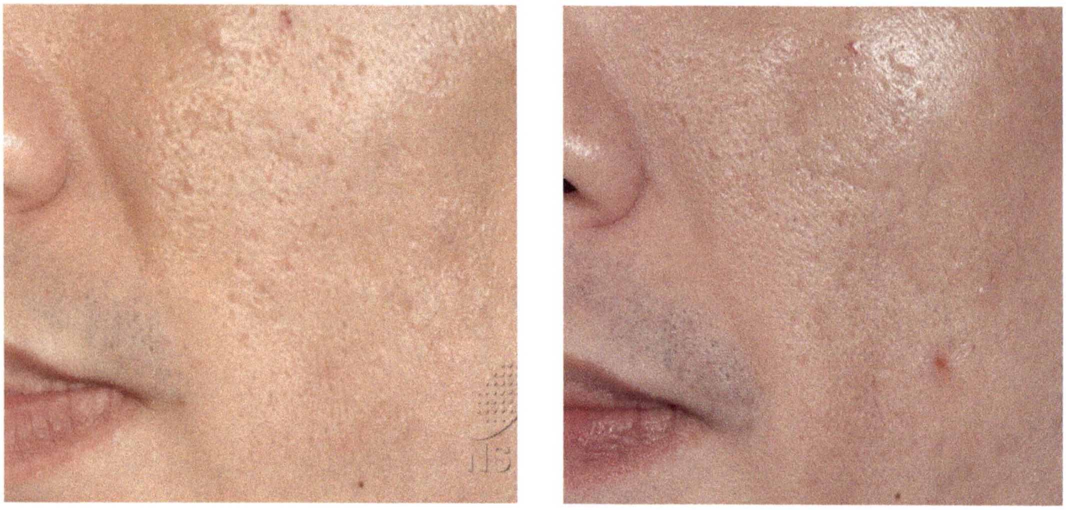

Before treatment. After treatment.

Figure 10.8.

A 38-year-old man with atrophic acne scars showing significant clinical improvement after 3 treatment sessions with the Mixto SX^{TM} fractional CO_2 laser. Treatment parameters used: 300 micron spot size, power 14–16 watts, index 6, treatment density 20%.

valaciclovir, or famciclovir, to prevent reactivation of the virus post treatment.

Treatment Protocols

The 2 key laser parameters influencing clinical outcomes are energy level and treatment density. Appropriate settings should be guided by recommendations made by the manufacturer of the specific device used. These guidelines are often updated as data from more clinical studies and experiences are available.

The depth of laser penetration is energy-dependent. Higher energy levels affect both depth of penetration as well as radial zone of thermal damage.[25,26] As such, the surface area finally treated is determined by the combined effect of energy level and treatment density.

In general, lower energy levels combined with higher treatment densities (20–40%) are employed to treat superficial problems such as fine rhytides and epidermal dyschromias. Higher energy levels coupled with lower treatment densities (15–20%) are employed to safely treat deeper problems such as moderate rhytides and acne scars. Lower energy levels coupled with lower treatment densities should be employed for off-face resurfacing.[27]

High energy levels coupled with high treatment densities run significant risks of causing bulk heating and should generally be avoided. Other pitfalls to avoid in treatment include poor lasering techniques, such as stacking of pulses or rapid application of laser passes before adequate skin cooling has occurred. These actions often result in bulk heating and its undesirable consequences.

Theoretically, the concomitant use of forced air cooling may reduce treatment efficacy. However, this concern has not been shown to be significant in NAFP, and forced air cooling is routinely used to improve patient comfort during treatment. On the other hand, the use of forced air cooling in AFP has not been well evaluated and, in the author's opinion, is generally not recommended.

FP is repeated 4–5 times at 4–8 weekly intervals. Clinical results are progressive, with optimal cosmetic improvement achieved in 3–6 months after the final treatment.

Preparation and Treatment

The way that the procedure is performed and the preparation involved will depend on the specific device used, e.g. the need for contact gels, cooling systems, optical dyes, topical anesthetics, etc.

As an illustration, we will describe the process involved with treatment using the Mixto SX™ Lasering fractional CO_2 laser. Topical anesthesia is applied to the skin under occlusion for 60–90 minutes before the procedure. The skin is cleansed with a mild cleanser and gently patted dry. The patient's eyes are protected using non-reflective goggles. Treatment within the orbital rim will further require the use of intra-ocular shields.

The procedure is performed using the fractional laser scanner, which is held away from the skin surface and does not come into contact with the skin. The spot size may be selected at 180 microns or 300 microns. The treatment area can be adjusted from 6 × 6 mm to 20 × 20 mm, with increments of 2 mm. The energy level is adjusted by setting the power and the treatment index that determines the pulse duration. Treatment density of 5–40% may be selected.

Suggested Mixto SX™ laser parameters are used for the following indications:

- Superficial dyschromias: 300 micron spot size, power 8–10 watts, index 6–8, treatment density 20–40%.
- Mild facial photaging: 300 micron spot size, power 8–10 watts, index 6–8, treatment density 20–40%.
- Moderate to severe facial photoaging: 300 micron spot size, power 10–16 watts, index 6, treatment density 20%. Alternatively, 180 micron spot size, power 8–10 watts, index 6–8, treatment density 20%.
- Acne scars: 300 micron spot size, power 10–16 watts, index 6, treatment density 20%. Alternatively, 180 micron spot size, power 8–10 watts, index 6–8, treatment density 20% may be used.
- Off-face resurfacing: 300 micron spot size, power 8–10 watts, index 6–8, treatment density 20%.

The laser spots are placed in 4 quadrants within the treatment area by a scanning algorithm that keeps the longest possible interval between two adjacent spots. This minimizes bulk heating and heat accumulation around the treated areas. A complete procedure consists of a single pass of the laser scanner, which places with precision micro-laser spots on the skin. Treatment of the entire face takes about 30 minutes. Mild to moderate pinprick pain that is well tolerated is felt.

Postoperative Care

There will be a burning sensation on the skin that lasts between 60 minutes and 6 hours immediately after treatment. To minimize discomfort and to reduce pain, patients may take paracetamol or non-steroidal anti-inflammatory drugs (NSAIDs). Cold compresses over the treatment area will also help minimize the discomfort.

Swelling may be managed by cold compresses and by avoiding strenuous activities for several days post treatment. The routine use of systemic or topical steroids to reduce post-treatment swelling is not recommended.

Treatment results in a bronzed appearance, similar to a darker tan, for the first week. Fine pixelated scabs will be formed by the skin as part of the normal healing process after AFP. Frequent use of a bland moisturizer such as aquaphor or vaseline will help the re-epithelialization process. With more aggressive treatment parameters, recovery may take longer.

Makeup can be used one day after NAFP but after AFP is best avoided until the scabs have fallen off.

Patients are advised to avoid sun exposure for at least three months. A sunscreen of SPF 30 or higher should be applied every day after the first week. Use of hydroquinone 2–4% starting one week after treatment may help reduce the incidence of PIH.

Side Effects and Complications

Post-inflammatory hyperpigmentation occurs in 5–10% of treated patients, especially in Fitzpatrick skin phototypes IV–VI, and may last several weeks to months. Treatment options to speed up resolution include topical bleaching agents (e.g. hydroquinone, kojic acid), tretinoin, glycolic acid products, and broad spectrum sunscreen to prevent further UV-light-induced melanin synthesis.

Acneiform eruptions occur in 2–4% of treated patients and is treated with a course of systemic tetracyclines, e.g. doxycyline 100 mg bid or erythromycin 500 mg bid for 6–12 weeks.

Reactivation of HSV occurs in 1–2% of treated patients and must be managed aggressively to prevent potential dissemination and subsequent scarring. This complication is largely preventable with the use of antiviral prophylaxis in patients with a past history of cold sores, especially if treatment involves the peri-oral region. The eruption of punctuate, painful erosions after treatment must alert the doctor to the likelihood of HSV reactivation. Systemic antivirals, e.g. valaciclovir 0.5 g bid, should be given immediately while awaiting results of confirmatory laboratory tests.

Conclusion

Fractional photothermolysis represents a significant advance in laser resurfacing by introducing a novel way of delivering laser energy to the skin in order to reap the benefits of conventional ablative laser resurfacing without its accompanying downtime and complications. The technology for FP is still evolving and being refined to further improve the benefit-to-risk ratio. Through the induction of strictly confined zones of thermal damage within the epidermis and dermis, FP triggers rapid epidermal repair and new dermal collagen formation. Additional esthetic and medical indications for FP are likely to be added to the current list as the benefits of FP are further explored.

References

1. Manstein D, Herron GS, Sink RK, *et al.* (2004) Fractional photothermolysis: a new concept for cutaneous remodeling using microscopic patterns of thermal injury. *Lasers Surg Med* **34**: 426–438.
2. Laubach H, Chan HH, Rius F, *et al.* (2006) Skin responses to fractional photothermolysis. *Lasers Surg Med* **38**: 142–149.
3. Hantash BM, Bedi VP, Sudireddy V, *et al.* (2006) Laser-induced transepidermal elimination of dermal content by fractional photothermolysis. *J Biomed Opt* **11**: 041115.
4. Walgrave S, Zelickson B, Childs J, *et al.* (2008) Pilot investigation of the correlation between histological and clinical effects of infrared fractional resurfacing lasers. *Dermatol Surg* **34**: 1443–1453.
5. Weiss R, Weiss M, Beasley K. (2008) Prospective split-face trial of a fixed spacing array computed scanned fractional CO_2 laser vs hand scanned 1550 nm fractional for rhytides. *Lasers Surg Med* **S20**: 31.
6. Lapidoth M, Yagima Odo ME, Odo LM. (2008) Novel use of erbium: YAG (2,940-nm) laser for fractional ablative photothermolysis in the treatment of photodamaged facial skin: a pilot study. *Dermatol Surg* **34**: 1048–1053.
7. Lomeo G, Cassuto DA, Scrimali L, *et al.* (2008) Er:YAG versus CO_2 ablative fractional resurfacing: a split face study. *Lasers Surg Med* **S20**: 30.
8. Alster TS, Tanzi EL, Lazarus M. (2007) The use of fractional laser photothermolysis for the treatment of atrophic scars. *Dermatol Surg* **33**: 295–299.
9. Lee HS, Lee JH, Ahn GY, *et al.* (2008) Fractional photothermolysis for the treatment of acne scars: a report of 27 Korean patients. *J Dermatol Treat* **19**: 45–49.

10. Chapas AM, Brightman L, Sukal S, *et al.* (2008) Successful treatment of acneiform scarring with CO_2 ablative fractional resurfacing. *Lasers Surg Med* **40**: 381–386.
11. Graber EM, Tanzi EL, Alster TS. (2008) Side effects and complications of fractional laser photothermolysis: experience with 961 treatments. *Dermatol Surg* **34**: 301–305.
12. Chan HH, Manstein D, Yu CS, *et al.* (2007) The prevalence and risk factors of post-inflammatory hyperpigmentation after fractional resurfacing in Asians. *Laser Surg Med* **39**: 381–385.
13. Jih MH, Goldberg LH, Kimyai-Asadi A. (2008) Fractional photothermolysis for photoaging of hands. *Dermatol Surg* **34**: 73–78.
14. Wanner M, Tanzi EL, Alster TS. (2007) Fractional photothermolysis: treatment of facial and nonfacial cutaneous photodamage with a 1550 nm erbium-doped fiber laser. *Dermatol Surg* **33**: 23–28.
15. Glaich AS, Rahman Z, Goldberg LH, *et al.* (2007) Fractional resurfacing for the treatment of hypopigmented scars: a pilot study. *Dermatol Surg* **33**: 289–294.
16. Tierney E, Mahmoud B, Srivastava D, *et al.* (2009) Treatment of surgical scars with fractional photothermolysis versus pulsed dye laser: randomized control trial. *Dermatol Surg* **35**: 1172–1180.
17. Rokhsar CK, Fitzpatrick RE. (2005) The treatment of melasma with fractional photothermolysis: a pilot study. *Dermatol Surg* **31**: 1645–1650.
18. Goldberg DJ, Berlin AL, Phelps R. (2008) Histologic and ultrastructural analysis of melasma after fractional resurfacing. *Lasers Surg Med* **40**: 134–138.
19. Naito SK. (2007) Fractional photothermolysis treatment for resistant melasma in Chinese females. *J Cosmet Laser Ther* **9**: 161–163.
20. Niwa AB, Mello AP, Torezan LA, *et al.* (2009) Fractional photothermolysis for the treatment of hypertrophic scars: clinical experience of eight cases. *Dermatol Surg* **35**: 773–777.
21. Behroozan DS, Goldberg LH, Glaich AS, *et al.* (2006) Fractional photothermolysis for treatment of poikiloderma of Civatte. *Dermatol Surg* **32**: 298–301.
22. Marra DE, Pourrabbani S, Fincher EF, *et al.* (2007) Fractional photothermolysis for the treatment of adult colloid milium. *Arch Dermatol* **143**: 572–574.
23. Lee HS, Won CH, Lee DH, *et al.* (2009) Treatment of melasma in Asian skin using a fractional 1550 nm laser: an open clinical study. *Dermatol Surg* **35**: 1499–1504.
24. Rahman Z, MacFalls H, Jiang K, *et al.* (2009) Fractional deep dermal ablation induces tissue tightening. *Lasers Surg Med* **41**: 78–86.
25. Bedi VP, Chan KF, Sink RK, *et al.* (2007) The effects of pulse energy variations on the dimensions of microscopic thermal treatment zones in nonablative fractional resurfacing. *Lasers Surg Med* **39**: 145–155.
26. Hantash BM, Bedi VP, Kapadia B, *et al.* (2007) *In vivo* histological evaluation of a novel ablative fractional resurfacing device. *Lasers Surg Med* **39**: 96–107.
27. Rahman Z, Alam M, Dover JS. (2006) Fractional laser treatment for pigmentation and texture improvement. *Skin Ther Lett* **11**: 7–11.

Chapter 11

Intense Pulsed Light Devices in the Asian Skin

Joyce Teng-Ee Lim*

Introduction

Intense pulsed light treatments (IPL) are safe and effective in treating a wide range of medical and esthetic skin conditions in Asian patients. An IPL device uses a high intensity pulsed light to target the skin chromophores (namely hemoglobin, melanin, and water) using the principle of selective photothermolysis as proposed by Anderson and Parrish.[1] It was first used as a medical device for treating vascular lesions.[2] Over the years, new indications were added and, today, IPL devices are used to treat a variety of skin conditions, including pigmented lesions, vascular lesions, poikiloderma of Civatte, photodamaged skin, hypertrichosis, and acne. It is most commonly used for photorejuvenation, as it improves skin tone, texture, and clarity with minimal downtime.

Intense Pulsed Light Devices

All IPL devices use an electrical capacitor bank, flashlamps, and wavelength filters to emit a high-intensity, polychromatic pulsed light that targets the various skin chromophores. Electrical energy from the capacitor bank passes through the xenon gas in the flashlamp to generate a polychromatic, pulsed high-intensity light in a broad wavelength spectrum of 515–1200 nm. There are second-generation IPL devices that use water to filter off the infrared part of the light spectrum, keeping the wavelength spectrum between 515–950 nm. This reduces the risk of epidermal damage and thus minimize the incidence of side effects. Patients with a darker skin tone, Fitzpatrick skin type V or VI,[3] have a higher risk of IPL-induced burns and using the narrower wavelength spectrum of 560–950 nm makes the IPL treatments safer.

There are various IPL devices in use and they can be grouped into two types depending on the beam profile (Fig. 11.1). The first-generation IPL devices produce a sigmoidal-shaped beam profile where the maximum energy is delivered within the first few milliseconds (the effective pulse) and this energy then decreases rapidly. The second-generation IPL devices have a larger electrical capacitor and give off a more constant train of energy, resulting in a flat-top or square-shaped beam profile where the effective energy is delivered over a longer period of time. This means that there is less fluctuation in the spectral distribution within a pulse and it is therefore safer, with less risk of side effects in treating Asian skin types.

All IPL devices differ in their cut-off filters, the pulse duration, the pulsing mode, and the fluence used. It is very difficult to compare the effectiveness of the various devices due to the diversity of these parameters. However, the general principles remain the same, which is to choose the appropriate cut-off filters or wavelength, the right pulse duration, and the optimal fluence and pulsing mode to treat a particular skin lesion and to adjust these parameters according to the skin response (Table 11.1).

*Consultant Dermatologist, Joyce Lim Skin and Laser Clinic, Paragon Medical Centre, Singapore.

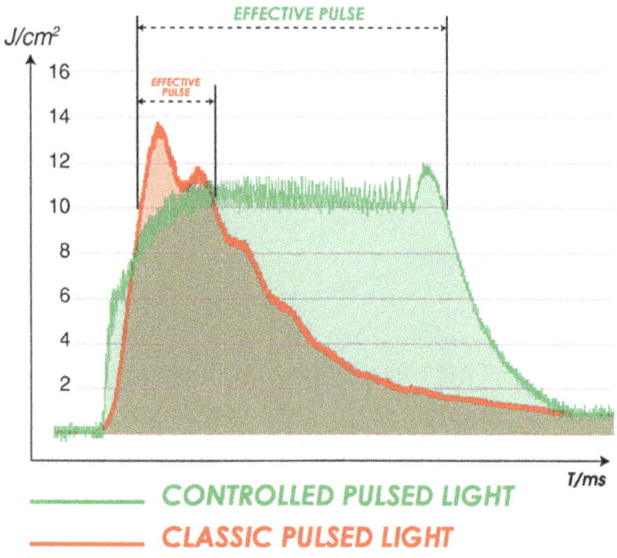

Figure 11.1.

The classic sigmoidal shaped beam profile and the square-shaped beam profile.

Table 11.1.

Treatment Parameters

1. Wavelength/cut-off filters: 420–1200 nm
2. Fluence
3. Pulse duration: 2–20 ms
4. Pulsing mode: single, double, triple

Various cut-off filters are used to obtain the wavelength spectrum for targeting the different skin chromophores. For instance, to treat pigmented lesions we use cut-off filters of 515–640 nm; for vascular lesions we use cut-off filters of 560–640 nm; and to remove hairs we use cut-off filters of 690–750 nm. Adjusting to the optimal wavelength spectrum using the different cut-off filters will allow for treating the different depths of the target structures and also for treating the different skin types. In general, a higher cut-off filter is used to treat deeper lesions and also for treating darker skin types (since higher filters reduce the absorption of melanin). We would choose a 515 nm filter to treat pigmented lesions in fair skin and a 560 nm filter to treat pigmented lesions in a darker skin type. We use a lower cut-off filter like 560 nm to treat bright red vessels and a higher filter like 590 nm to treat blue vessels.

Pulse duration is set in milliseconds (ms) from 0.5–88 ms, less than the thermal relaxation time of the target structure, based on the principle of selective photothermolysis.[1] A longer pulse duration is used when treating darker skin types and in treating larger structures like larger vessels or hairs.

The amount of energy per unit area applied to the skin during treatment and the amount of heat built up in the skin is determined by the fluence. Darker targets absorb more energy and will reach higher temperatures. Therefore darker lesions require less fluence than lighter colored lesions to reach the same therapeutic level. The fluence can be delivered in a single pulse or in multiple pulses. When using high fluence and/or treating Asian skin, it is safer to split the fluence into multiple pulses, and the intervals between the individual pulses can be set at between 1–300 ms. This delay allows the epidermal cells and smaller vessels to cool down between pulses while heat is retained in the larger vessels and hair follicles. When treating Asian patients, choose the lowest fluence that gives the desired tissue response and use double- or triple-pulsing to reduce the risk of side effects.

Indications for IPL Treatment

IPL devices are versatile and can be used to treat a wide range of skin conditions. (Table 11.2).

Pre-Treatment Counseling

This includes a discussion of the various treatment options, explanation of the procedure, the risk of side effects and complications as well as the expected degree of improvement. Patients must have realistic

Table 11.2.

Skin Conditions Amendable to IPL Treatments

1. *Acne*
2. *Vascular lesions*
   Telangiectasias
   Rosacea
   Port wine stains
   Erythema
   Flushing
   Venous lakes
3. *Pigmented lesions*
   Freckles
   Melasma
   Solar lentigines
4. *Photodamaged skin — facial and non-facial*
5. *Poikiloderma of Civatte*
6. *Hair removal*

expectations as the aim is to improve the skin condition and sometimes it is not possible to completely eradicate it. Multiple sessions are often necessary and results vary with each individual. Patients with Fitzpatrick skin types V and VI are often offered other treatment options as the risk of side effects are higher with IPL treatments.

The physician must be certain of the diagnosis and decide whether IPL is the best choice of treatment. A suspected malignant lesion should not be treated but instead a biopsy must be done. Relative contraindications include pregnancy, breast feeding, the intake of any photosensitizing medications, the presence of diseases that tend to worsen on sun exposure, and a recent suntan. Patients are advised to avoid sun exposure, tanning beds, and tanning creams for 2–3 weeks prior to treatment. If sun exposure is unavoidable, the fluence has to be set lower.

Patient Preparation

The area to be treated is cleaned with a mild cleanser. Topical anesthesia, e.g. EMLA®, a eutectic mixture of lidocaine 2.5% and prilocaine 2.5%, may be used to alleviate discomfort. The topical anesthetic is removed before starting treatment.

The IPL Procedure

IPL procedures are safe and effective if performed properly. As there is a great variety of devices, physicians must know their own machine well and know the optimal parameters for treating a particular skin lesion in different skin types.

Epidermal skin cooling is important, especially when treating Asian patients. Cooling is provided by the contact cooling plate as well as the chilled coupling gel. In most IPL devices, the temperature of the contact cooling plate can be adjusted. The amount of cooling required depends on the depth of the skin lesion and the Fitzpatrick skin type. Darker skin types require more cooling for deeper lesions.

A coupling gel is applied on the skin and this may be chilled. The gel must be adequately layered across the treatment area. Before starting, protective goggles must be worn. Use the correct cut-off filter to give the desired wavelength spectrum, key in the correct pulse duration, fluence, and pulsing sequence. The handpiece must be cleaned before it is placed with the cooling plate perpendicular and in full contact with the skin. Allow a few seconds before depressing the switch, to cool the skin surface. In order to treat small areas, use a smaller spot adapter or a perforated plastic shield with varying aperture sizes, or simply use a piece of nonabsorbent white paper with an area corresponding to the lesion size punched out.

It is important to do a test spot during the first session, especially when the patient is of Fitzpatrick skin type IV or V. Test spots should be done at an inconspicuous site. Wait a few minutes to see the skin response (Table 11.3) and then adjust the treatment parameters accordingly. Always begin with a lower fluence and assess the response before increasing the

Table 11.3.

Skin Response to IPL

Desired response	
1.	Darkening of freckles or brown spots
2.	Reduction of caliber of blood vessels
3.	Dark blue or gray discoloration of larger blood vessels
4.	Mild erythema within a few seconds
Undesired response	
1.	Prolonged erythema
2.	Swelling, urticaria, blisters
3.	Crusting

fluence or decreasing the pulse duration. It is a good practice to do test spots when treating different parts of the body as the skin response to IPL varies in different parts of the body.

Once you have the desired treatment response, treat the whole area with minimum overlap or at most a 10% overlap, matching the "trailing edge" of the next treatment spot to the "leading edge" of the previous treatment area. During treatment, do not stack pulses even if you do not see a response. If needed, you can treat the same area later during the second pass. When treating over bony areas or nonfacial areas, reduce the treatment fluence by 20%. Treat the entire face, including the lower eyelids and the area just below the jaw line. The upper eyelids are generally not treated.

Post-IPL Care

Generally, IPL treatments do not need any aftercare other than using a sunblock. If the skin feels tight or looks red, a cool compress or ice pack may be used immediately after the procedure. If blisters or crusting is seen, patients should be given a topical antibiotic. Makeup and sunblock may be applied right after treatment. Excessive sun exposure should be avoided and treatments are usually repeated at 4–6 week intervals.

Pigmented Lesions

Although Q-switched lasers are effective in treating pigmented lesions, IPL has a place in treating the Asian patient as it is safe and effective. For Fitzpatrick skin types II–III, it is safe to use cut-off filters of 515–560 nm, whereas for skin types IV–V, a higher cut-off filter of 560–640 nm is preferred.

Freckles (Ephelides)

IPL is effective and safe for the treatment of freckles in Asians. Huang *et al.*[4] treated 36 patients with freckles using the Vasculight™ (ESC/Sharplan, Yokneam, Israel). IPL treatment was administered every four weeks using cut-off filters ranging from 550 to 590 nm, with a fluence of 25–35 J/cm^2, with single- or double-pulse illumination and a pulse width of 4.0 ms. By the end of the study, physicians' assessment was excellent or good for 86.1% of the subjects, while 91.7% of the patients reported that they were extremely or very satisfied. There were relatively few adverse effects. One patient had hypopig-mentation that spontaneously resolved within one month. Erythema and pain were transient, disappearing after one or two days. All evidence of crusting had disappeared within one week. A mean of 1.47 sessions was required to treat the freckles.

A study by Negishi *et al.*[5] who treated Japanese patients with freckles, showed that IPL is effective and safe with minimal side effects.

Solar Lentigines

Solar lentigines may be treated with cryosurgery, electrosurgery, or lasers. IPL is also effective in treating solar lentigines (Fig. 11.2). Kawada *et al.*[6] treated 60 patients with solar lentigines and ephelides. The NatuLight™ (Lumenis, Tokyo) was used with 560 nm cut-off filter, fluence 20–24 J/cm^2, pulse duration 2.6–5.0, double or triple pulses and pulse delay 20 ms.

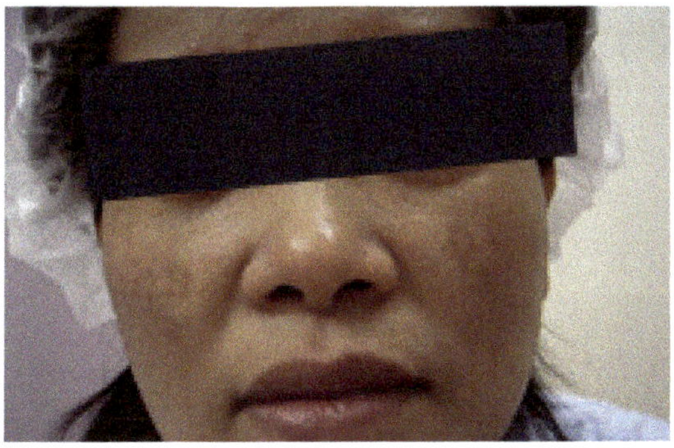

Before treatment.

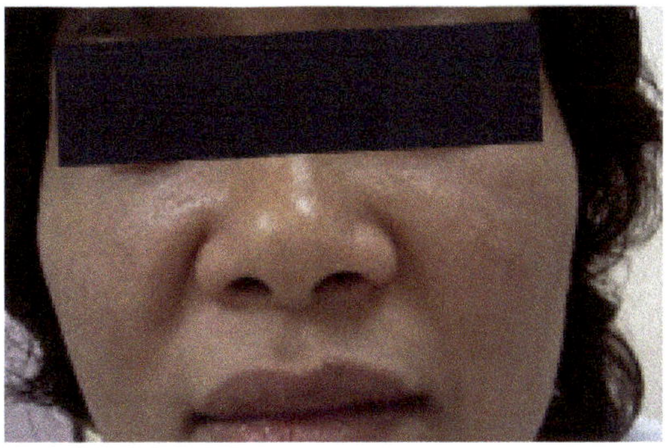

After 3 treatments at monthly intervals with the Medilux™ (Palomer Medical Technologies, USA) using the Lux G handpiece: wavelength spectrum 500–670 nm, fluence 21 J/cm^2, spot size 12 x 12 mm, pulse duration 20 ms, showing excellent improvement. Clinical endpoint: darkening of lesion and perilesional erythema. (Courtesy of Tay YK, FRCP, Singapore).

Figure 11.2.

Lentigines.

After 3–5 treatments, 16% of patients had an improvement of more than 75%, while 40% of patients had an improvement of more than 50% in their solar lentigines. Patients with small plaques of solar lentigines responded well, whereas patients with large plaques showed poor response.

In his study, Bjerring *et al.*[7] was able to treat solar lentigines in a single treatment with some success. He used the Ellipse Flex™ (Danish Dermatologic Development) with wavelength spectrum 400–720 nm, fluence 10–20 J/cm^2, spot size 10–48 mm, pulse duration 7 ms, double pulse with a pulse delay of 25 ms. Two months after a single treatment, there was evidence of pigment reduction in 96% of patients (from close-up photography) and an average clearance of 74.2%.

Melasma

Topical therapy remains the gold standard in the treatment of melasma. However, it is difficult to clear melasma with topical treatments alone, and IPL treatments are often added (Fig. 11.3). Li *et al.*[8] studied the efficacy and safety of IPL treatments in treating melasma in Chinese patients using the Lumenis One™ (Lumenis Inc, Santa Clara, California). Treatment parameters used were cut-off filters 560/590 nm with double pulse, or cut-off filters 590/615/640 nm with triple pulse and a fluence of 13–17 J/cm^2, pulse duration of 3–4 ms, and pulse delay of 25–40 ms. Eighty-nine patients were treated for four sessions at 3-weekly intervals. Dermatological assessment at the end of the study showed 77.5% of the patients having a 51–100% improvement, while 70.8% of the patients had 50% or more improvement. There was a decrease in melasma area and severity index (MASI) from 15.2 to 4.5.

Wang *et al.*[9] treated 17 patients from Taiwan with refractory melasma with IPL at 4-weekly intervals for four sessions. Melasma improved by 39.8% compared to only 11.6% improvement in the control group. Two patients in the intense pulsed light group experienced transient, post-inflammatory hyperpigmentation, and

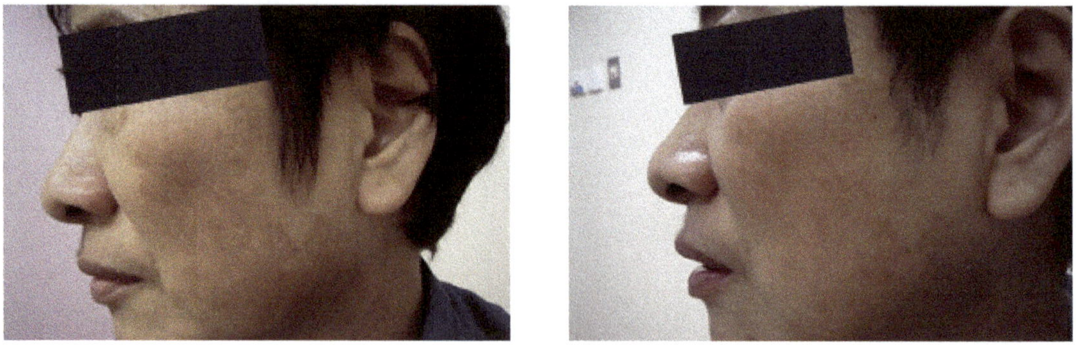

Before treatment.

After 4 treatments at monthly intervals with the Medilux™ (Palomar) using the Lux Y handpiece: wavelength spectrum 525–1200 nm, fluence 15 J/cm^2, spot size 16 x 46 mm, pulse duration 40 ms showing moderate improvement. Clinical endpoint: mild erythema. (Courtesy of Tay YK, FRCP, Singapore).

Figure 11.3.

Melasma.

partial repigmentation was noted 24 weeks after the last treatment session.

Negishi *et al.*[5] treated four patients with melasma with IPL and showed improvement in pigmentation and texture. No mention was made about the type of melasma. Patients were on bleaching agents after the third treatment session and there was no control in this study.

Vascular Lesions

IPL is effective in coagulating vessels that are 60–500 μm without ecchymosis. It is used successfully to treat a variety of vascular lesions, namely telangiectasias, rosacea, port wine stains, angiomas, and spider nevi. A dark blue or gray discoloration is seen immediately after the IPL treatment.

Facial Telangiectasias

Facial telangiectasias may be treated with lasers, e.g. the pulsed dye laser or the pulsed potassium-titanyl-phosphate (KTP) laser, with good results. However, Bjerring *et al.*[10] showed that IPL can also treat facial telangiectasia effectively and safely. Using the Ellipse Flex™ (Danish Dermatologic Development) with wavelength spectrum of 555–950 nm, fluence 10–26 J/cm^2, spot size 10–48 mm, and pulse duration 10–30 ms, 24 patients were treated at monthly intervals for a total of 2–3 treatments. Of the patients treated, 79.2% obtained more than 50% reduction in the number of vessels and 37.5% obtained 75–100% reduction two months after their last treatment. The procedure was effective and safe with minimal side effects, including moderate erythema and edema. There were no scars or pigmentary changes.

In a larger study, Retamar *et al.*[11] treated 140 patients with facial telangiectasias. They found IPL treatments to be safe and effective. They found 94 (67.1%) patients responded with excellent results (80–100% clearance), 43 (30.7%) with good results (40–80% clearance), and 3 (2.1%) with poor results (< 40% clearance). Side effects were minimal and transient. An earlier study by Angermeier,[12] who treated 153 patients using the PhotoDerm VL™

(Lumenis Ltd Yokneam, Israel), with wavelength spectrum of 550–570 nm, fluence 36–45 J/cm^2, pulse duration 2.5–6 ms, and pulse delay 20–30 ms, also had good results with 75–100% clearance of telangiectasias after 1–4 treatments.

Nyman *et al.*[13] compared the efficacy and safety of IPL treatments, using the Ellipse Flex™ (Danish Dermatologic Development) with the long-pulsed dye laser (LPDL), in the treatment of telangiectasias that occurred after radiotherapy for breast cancer. The treatment parameters used were wavelength spectrum of 530–750 nm or 555–950 nm, fluence of 8–20 J/cm^2, spot size 10 × 48 mm, and a pulse duration of 10–20 ms. He treated 13 patients in a split-lesion study, for three sessions at 6-weekly intervals. Patients were evaluated three months after the last session. The LPDL was more effective in clearing the telangiectasia: 90% of vessels cleared with the LPDL compared to 50% with the IPL, and more patients preferred the LPDL.

Leg Telangiectasias

IPL treatment is useful only for treating leg telangiectasia if the vessel caliber is < 1 mm diameter. In a multicenter study, Goldman *et al.*[14] treated 159 patients with the PhotoDerm VL™ (Lumenis Ltd Yokneam, Israel). There was a 90% clearance rate with vessels < 0.2 mm diameter and a clearance rate of 80% with vessels measuring 0.2–1 mm diameter. Similar results were also seen by Schroeter *et al.*[15] in their multicenter study of 40 patients. They had clearance rates of 92.1%, 80%, and 81% for vessels of 0.2 mm, 0.2–0.5 mm, and 0.5–1 mm diameter.

Leg veins of >1 mm diameter are better treated with sclerotherapy or the long-pulsed Nd:YAG laser. Fodor *et al.*[16] compared the IPL treatment of leg veins with that of Nd:YAG laser treatment in a prospective side-to-side study. Patients with leg veins <1 mm diameter were more satisfied with the IPL treatments. However, they found that leg veins >1 mm diameter were better treated with the Nd:YAG laser, although patients found the laser treatments more painful. Sadick,[17] in an earlier study, suggested treating red telangiectasias with a diameter of <1 mm with the IPL, while treating blue vessels with a diameter >1 mm with the long-pulsed Nd:YAG laser. He obtained significant clearance rates of 75–100% in 80% of the patients six months after the end of the treatment using this approach.

Rosacea

IPL is effective in treating the flushing, redness and telangiectasias seen in erythemato-telangiectatic rosacea. Results are comparable to those obtained with the pulsed dye laser. Schroeter *et al.*[18] treated facial telangiectasias in 60 patients with rosacea, using the Vasculight™ (Lumenis, Israel) with 515–1200 nm wavelength spectrum, fluence 25–35 J/cm^2, and pulse duration 4.3–6.5 ms. A mean clearance rate of 77.8% after an average of 4.1 treatments per area was achieved, based on both clinical and photographic evaluation. The clearance was maintained during the long follow-up period of 12–99 months (average 51.6 months). Only 4 of the 508 treated areas had a recurrence. Side effects were minimal.

Another study by Papageorgiou *et al.*[19] also confirmed the effectiveness of IPL in treating rosacea. The authors used the Quantum SR™ (Lumenis, Israel) with 560–1200 nm wavelength spectrum, spot size 34 × 8 mm, fluence 24–32 J/cm^2, and double pulsing. Thirty-four patients were treated for a total of four treatments at 3-weekly intervals. Erythema improved by 46% and telangiectasias by 55%. The severity of rosacea was reduced on average by 3.5 points on a 10-point visual analog scale. Follow-up at six months showed the results were maintained. Side effects were minimal and self-limiting.

The effectiveness of IPL in treating rosacea was compared with the pulsed dye laser by Neuhaus *et al.*[20] They treated 29 patients with erythemo-telangiectatic rosacea in a single-blind, split-face trial, using a spot size of 10 mm, fluence 7 J/cm^2, pulse duration 6 ms for the pulsed dye laser and a cut-off filter of 560 nm, fluence 25 J/cm^2, pulse train 2.4 and 6 ms, and a pulse delay of 15 ms for the IPL. Each patient had three treatments at monthly intervals. Both IPL and pulsed dye laser significantly reduced the cutaneous erythema, telangiectasia, and symptoms. There was no significant difference between the IPL and the pulsed dye laser treatments in terms of efficacy and side effects.

Port Wine Stains

The pulsed dye laser is the treatment of choice for port wine stains. However, IPL has also been used successfully in treating port wine stains. Ho *et al.*[21] treated 22 Chinese patients with port wine stains using the Multilight™ (ESC Medical Systems Ltd, Yokneam, Israel) with cut-off filters of 550, 570, and 590 nm, with a double or triple pulse. Each patient received 3–8 treatment sessions. More than 90% of patients had more than 25% clearance, 40% of patients had more than 50% clearance, and 9% of the patients were able to achieve more than 75% clearance. The only two patients with less than 25% clearing had nodular port wine stains and no patient was able to achieve complete clearance. The procedures were well tolerated. One patient developed blisters and six patients had swelling for more than 24 hours. These resolved within one week without leaving permanent marks. They were followed up for 12–27 months, and there were no long-term complications.

In a multicenter study, Raulin *et al.*[22] showed that IPL treatments can clear or lighten port wine stains using the PhotoDerm™ (Lumenis, Israel). They used cut-off filters of 515, 550, and 570 nm, fluence 20–70 J/cm^2, pulse duration 2.5–5 ms, and pulse mode of 1–3. They treated 37 patients with therapy-resistant port wine stains as well as those with purple and hypertrophic lesions. They achieved complete clearance of pink lesions after an average of four sessions. Very dark purple lesions were lightened by 70–99% after an average of four sessions.

Bjerring *et al.*[23] treated 15 patients with pulsed-dye-laser-resistant port wine stains with the Ellipse Flex™ (Danish Dermatologic Development), with wavelength spectrum of 555–950 nm, fluence 13–22 J/cm^2, spot size 10–48 mm, and pulse duration 8–30 ms. Each lesion was treated 4 times. There was a lightening of more than 50% in 7 out of 15 patients. Side effects were uncommon, with 9% having hypopigmentation, 3% having hyperpigmentation, and none developing any scar. Ozdemir *et al.*[24] also showed that IPL is effective for port wine stains.

Faurschou *et al.*[25] compared the IPL treatments using the Starlux™ (Palomar Medical Technologies, USA) with that of the pulsed dye laser in a side-by-side trial in 20 patients with port wine stains (12 had previous treatments while 8 had not). The IPL parameters used were cut-off filters of 500–670 nm and 870–1400 nm, fluence 7–14 J/cm^2, and pulse duration 5–10 ms. Both the IPL and pulsed dye laser were able to lighten the port wine stain. The group treated by the pulsed dye laser did better, with 65% having clinical improvement compared to 30% in the IPL group. In another study, Babilas *et al.*[26] compared the efficacy of an IPL device with two different pulsed dye lasers, the flashlamp-pumped pulsed dye laser (FPDL) and the long-pulsed tunable dye laser (LPTDL), in treating port wine stains. They showed that the IPL device was better in treating port wine stains compared to the FPDL and as effective as the LPTDL.

McGill *et al.*[27] compared an IPL device, Lumina™ (Lynton Lasers, UK), with a pulsed dye laser, an alexandrite, a KTP, and a Nd:YAG laser in treating treatment-resistant port wine stains in 18 patients, using all devices in treating parts of the lesion. They used wavelength spectrum 550–1100 nm, fluence 28–34 J/cm^2, double pulses with 10 ms delay. The alexandrite laser was the most effective (10 patients improved), while the KTP and Nd:YAG lasers were the least effective (two patients improved with each device). The IPL device improved the port wine stains in six patients and the pulsed dye laser in five patients.

Hemangiomas

Most hemangiomas will resolve spontaneously and treatments are started if the growth is rapid, if the hemangioma interferes with vital functions, or if there are complications like infection or ulceration. The treatment of choice is the pulsed dye laser. Angermeier[12] used the PhotoDerm™ (Lumenis, Israel) with cut-off filters 550, 570, 590 nm, fluence 36–45 J/cm^2, pulse duration 2.5–6 ms, pulse delay 20–30 ms, and triple-pulse mode to treat 45 patients with centrofacial hemangiomas. Each patient had 1–4 treatments, and there was 75–100% clearance of the hemangioma.

Poikiloderma of Civatte

IPL treatments can improve the erythema and hyperpigmentation associated with poikiloderma of Civatte. Weiss *et al.*[28] used the PhotoDerm VL™ (Lumenis, Israel) with cut-off filters 515, 550, 570 nm, fluence 20–24 J/cm^2, pulse duration 2–4 ms, pulse delay 10 ms, single or double pulse to treat 135 patients with poikiloderma of Civatte. One hundred and eleven patients (82%) achieved 75–100% clearance after three treatments. Goldman *et al.*[29] achieved 50–75% improvement after an average of 2.8 treatments using cut-off filters 550, 570, 590 nm, fluence 22–60 J/cm^2, pulse duration 3–6 ms, and pulse delay 10–30 ms in a single-, double-, or triple-pulsed mode.

Photorejuvenation

Skin aging consists of pigmentary alterations, e.g. lentigines and melasma, and vascular alterations, e.g. telangiectasias, diffuse redness, and wrinkles. IPL treatments are commonly used for skin rejuvenation as they are effective in removing the pigmentary and vascular alterations and there is little downtime. Negishi *et al.*[30] did skin biopsies from the temples of Japanese patients three weeks after a series of five IPL treatments spaced three weeks apart, and showed significant collagen deposition just below the skin. Bitter[31] compared skin biopsies taken from the forehead before and four weeks after 4 full-face IPL treatments and showed that new collagen was seen in both the papillary and reticular dermis. There was a resolution in the superficial dermal inflammatory infiltrate. Feng *et al.*[32] studied skin biopsies taken from Chinese patients before and after IPL treatments and showed an increase in type 1 and 3 collagen and more orderly arranged elastic fibers. Electron microscopy showed increased fibroblast activity and the collagen fibers were neatly rearranged within the stroma.

Bitter[31] was one of the first to use the IPL device for photorejuvenation. He used the Vasculight™ (Lumenis, CA) to treat the whole face, and each patient had four treatments at 3–4 weekly intervals. There was an improvement of 10–90% in rhytides, skin texture, pore size, and telangiectasia. There were minimal side effects: transient erythema and rare blisters — all resolved spontaneously.

Negishi *et al.*[30] treated Japanese patients with skin types IV and V with the Vasculight™ (Lumenis, CA) and achieved an improvement of 56–100% in pigmentation, telangiectasias, and skin texture in 66–91% of their patients. In another study, they had a 60% improvement in over 80% of their patients.[5] Side effects were transient erythema and blistering. There were no pigmentary changes.

Li *et al.*[33] treated 152 Chinese patients with photodamaged skin, using the Lumenis One™ (Lumenis, CA), with wavelength spectrum of 515–1200 nm, fluence 11–20 J/cm^2, double or triple pulse, pulse duration 2.5–4 ms, and delay 20–40 ms. Each patient had four treatments 3–4 weeks apart. Dermatologist assessment showed a decrease of 2–3 grades in 139 of 153 patients (91.44%). Patient assessment showed an overall excellent or good improvement in 136 of 152 patients (89.47%). The mean skin melanin index (MI) and erythema index (EI) decreased with each session.

Adverse effects seen were mild pain and transient erythema.

Bjerring *et al.*[34] compared the safety and clinical efficacy of two different wavelength spectra (555–950 nm VL or 530–750 nm PR) in the treatment of 35 patients with photodamaged skin. They used the Ellipse Flex™ (Danish Dermatologic Development) with a fluence of 6–20 J/cm^2, spot size 10–48 mm, pulse duration 2 × 2.5 ms, and pulse delay 10 or 8–20 ms. They found that the higher wavelength spectrum VL filter was better for clearance of pigmentation, whereas the PR filter was better for clearing telangiectasias and diffuse erythema. Fair to excellent results were seen in 66.7% treated with the PR filter, and 76.2% with the VL filter. Side effects of swelling and erythema were higher (66%) with the PR filter compared to 33% with the VL filter. When treating Asian skin to reduce the risk of side effects, the VL filter is often used.

The efficacy and safety of IPL treatments for photodamaged skin were compared with the long-pulsed tunable dye laser (LPDL) by Jorgensen *et al.*[35] in a split-face study using the Ellipse Flex™ (Danish Dermatologic Development) with a fluence of 6–20 J/cm^2, spot size 10–48 mm, pulse duration 2 × 2.5 ms, and pulse delay 10 or 8–20 ms. Twenty women of Fitzpatrick skin types I–III were treated, each having three treatments at 3-weekly intervals. The LPDL achieved better clearance of vessels and was less painful. Both the LPDL and the IPL had equal improvements in pigmentation and skin texture, but in both there was no reduction of rhytides.

Kono *et al.*[36] did a similar comparison in a split-face study using the IPL device Smooth pulsed light™ (Palomar Corporation, USA) and the LPDL in treating 10 Asian patients. Each patient had six treatment sessions using IPL wavelength spectrum of 470–1400 nm, fluence 27–40 J/cm^2, and pulse duration 20 ms. Patients were evaluated three months after the last treatment. Lentigines improved by 81.1% with the LPDL and 62.3% with the IPL. Neither device improved wrinkles and both were safe with no scarring or pigmentary changes.

Hair Removal

IPL devices are commonly used to remove hairs. There are several controlled studies that document the effectiveness of IPL in hair removal, especially in patients with fair skin and dark hairs. Feng *et al.*[32] treated 18 Chinese patients with Fitzpatrick skin types III–V and dark hairs. They studied the efficacy and effectiveness of the Lumenis One™ (Lumenis, Santa Clara, CA) using wavelength spectrum 550–1200 nm, fluence of 14–22 J/cm^2, pulse duration of 3–4 ms, and pulse delay of 25–40 ms in removing axillary hair in 13 patients and upper lip hair in five patients. Each patient had four treatments at 4–6 week intervals. They achieved an average hair reduction of 49.9% after the first session, 58.6% after the second session, 79.3% after the third sessions, and 83.8% after the last session. They found the IPL treatments to be safe and without significant side effects. Unfortunately, patients were not followed up long enough to see if there was any hair regrowth.

Cameron *et al.*[37] compared the efficacy of an IPL device, the Lumina™ (Lynton Lasers, UK) with a diode laser (Lightsheer EC™, Lumenis, USA) in a split-face study. They treated nine patients using wavelength spectrum 625–1100 nm, 32 J/cm^2, pulse train 8 × 4 ms, and total train time of 95 ms. Each patient had three treatments at 6-week intervals. The average hair counts were reduced by 75% with the laser and 50% with the IPL. Patients experienced more pain and inflammation on the laser-treated side. However, five patients preferred the laser treatments, while two preferred the IPL treatments.

Another spilt-face study by McGill *et al.*[38] compared the IPL device, Lumina™ (Lynton Lasers, UK) with an alexandrite laser, the GentleLase™ (Candela, USA). Thirty-eight women with polycystic ovary syndrome were treated with a wavelength spectrum of 650–1100 nm, 16–42 J/cm^2, 3 pulses of 55 ms, with pulse delay 20 ms. The alexandrite laser was more effective in hair reduction at 1, 3, and 6 months, and the median hair-free intervals was longer, at seven weeks for the laser compared with two weeks for the

IPL treatments. Other authors[39,40] have also compared the IPL treatments with lasers (diode, alexandrite) and found laser hair removal to be more effective and the hair-free intervals longer.

A study by Bjerring *et al.*[41] however, showed that IPL treatments were four times more effective in hair removal than the ruby laser. In their study they treated 31 patients in a split-face study comparing the Ellipse Relax Light 1000™ (Danish Dermatologic Development), using wavelength spectrum of 600–950 nm, fluence of 18.5 J/cm^2, spot size 10 × 48 mm, and a ruby laser Epitouch™ (Sharplan, ESC Israel).

Paradoxical hypertrichosis has been reported after IPL treatments. It tends to occur in patients with darker skin types and those with fine hairs prior to treatment.[42] This is seen most commonly in the low maxillary area, the neck, the lateral cheeks, and the chin in young women. It can occur within and outside the treatment areas. The incidence varies from 1–10.5%.[42–44] The mechanism of this is unclear and is thought to be due to subtherapeutic thermal energy applied to the hair follicles.

Acne Vulgaris

IPL treatments have been used for treating inflammatory and noninflammatory acne and results have not been consistent. Chang *et al.*[45] treated 30 female patients with mild to moderate acne in a split-face study, where one half of the face was treated with benzoyl peroxide gel alone and the other half of the face was treated with benzoyl peroxide gel plus IPL, using the Ellipse Flex™ (Danish Dermatologic Development) with a wavelength spectrum 530–750 nm, fluence of 7.5–8 J/cm^2, spot size 10–48 mm, pulse duration 2 × 2.5 ms, and pulse delay 10 ms. Each patient had three sessions of IPL at 3-weekly intervals. IPL did not improve the acne but it improved the red macules, the pigmentary changes, and the skin tone.

IPL is often used with photodynamic therapy (PDT) to treat acne. Yeung *et al.*[46] treated 30 Asian patients with skin type IV or V, using the Ellipse Flex™ (Danish Dermatologic Development) for four sessions at 3-weekly intervals. Patients were randomized to have split-face treatment, with either methyl aminolevulinate (MAL) PDT-IPL, IPL alone, or control. They found that the PDT-IPL- and IPL-treated sides showed significant reduction in the noninflammatory lesions compared to the control side but there were no significant differences between the two treated groups. However, 25% of patients in the PDT-IPL group withdrew from the study because of side effects. There were no significant differences in the treated side (either PDT-IPL or IPL) compared to the control side for reduction of the inflammatory lesions.

Side Effects and Complications

Side effects are generally uncommon unless the fluence is too high or the pulse duration too narrow.

The commonest side effects are erythema and swelling that last for 2–48 hours. Blisters and crusting can occur and patients are advised not to pick at the scabs to prevent scarring. A bland ointment like vaseline or a topical antibiotic like mupirocin can be used on the crusts. Transient purpura, crusting, hyper- and hypopigmentation are more common in dark-skinned individuals or tanned skin.

Side effects are more common in removing unwanted hair than for other indications. The common side effects are transient crusting, blisters, hyperpigmentation (Fig. 11.4), or hypopigmentation. Scarring after IPL is rare. Asian patients with Fitzpatrick skin types V or VI have a higher risk of burns and hyperpigmentation when IPL is used for hair removal. For such patients, laser hair removal should be the treatment of choice. If IPL treatment is used, then a higher cut-off filter and lower fluence should be used.

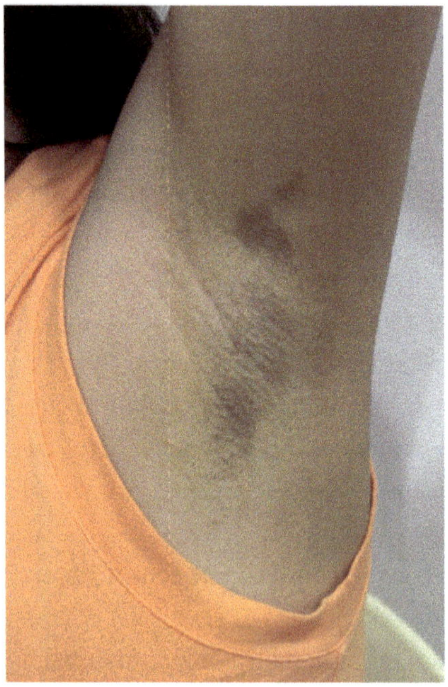

Figure 11.4.

Post-inflammatory hyperpigmentation after IPL for hair removal.

Dyschromasia of the upper eyelids with bilateral ocular iritis has been reported after IPL treatment of the eyelids without the use of eye shields.[47] This rare side effect serves to remind us of the importance of proper eye protection during IPL treatment

Conclusion

Intense pulsed light treatments are effective in treating a wide variety of pigmentary lesions, vascular lesions, photodamaged skin, and hypertrichosis in Asian patients with miminal side effects. As Asian patients have higher epidermal melanin content, the risk of side effects is higher. To minimize potential side effects and complications, always do a test spot and, if necessary, use a higher cut-off filter and lower fluence delivered in double or triple pulses.

References

1. Anderson RR, Parrish JA. (1983) Selective photothermolysis: precise microsurgery by selective absorption of pulsed radiation. *Science* **220**: 524–527.
2. Muhlbauer W, Nath G, Kreitmair A. (1976) Treatment of capillary hemangiomas and nevi flammei with light. *Langenbecks Arch Chir* (Suppl.), 91–94.
3. Fitzpatrick TB. (1988) The validity and practicality of sun-reactive skin types I through VI. *Arch Dermatol* **124**: 869–871.
4. Huang YL, Liao YL, Lee SH, *et al.* (2002) Intense Pulse light for the treatment of freckles in Asian skin. *Dermatol Surg* **28**: 1007–1012.
5. Negishi K, Tezuka Y, Kushikata N, *et al.* (2001) Photorejuvenation for Asian skin by intense pulsed light. *Dermatol Surg* **27**: 627–632.
6. Kawada A, Shiraishi H, Asai M, *et al.* (2002) Clinical improvement of solar lentigines/ephelides with an intense pulsed light source. *Dermatol Surg* **28**: 504–508.
7. Bjerring P, Christiansen K. (2000) Intense pulsed light source for treatment of small melanocytic nevi and solar lentigines. *J Cutan Laser Ther* **2**: 177–181.
8. Li YH, Chen JZ, Wei HC, *et al.* (2008) Efficacy and safety of intense pulsed light in the treatment of Chinese patients. *Dermatol Surg* **34**: 693–700.
9. Wang CC, Hui CY, Sue YM, *et al.* (2004) Intense pulsed light for the treatment of refractory melasma in Asian persons. *Dermatol Surg* **30**: 1196–1200.
10. Bjerring P, Christiansen K, Troilius A. (2001) Intense pulsed light source for treatment of facial telangiectasias. *J Cosmetic Laser Ther* **3**: 169–173.
11. Retamar RA, Chames C, Pellerano G. (2004) Treatment of linear and spider telangiectasia with an intense pulsed light source. *J Cosmet Dermatol* **3**: 187–190.
12. Angermeier MC. (1999) Treatment of facial vascular lesions with intense pulsed light. *J Cutan Laser Ther* **1**: 95–100.
13. Nymann P, Hedelund L, Haedersdal M. (2009) Intense pulsed light vs long pulse dye laser treatment of telangiectasia after radiotherapy for breast cancer: a randomised split-lesion trial of two different treatments. *Br J Dermatol* **160**: 1237–1241.
14. Goldman MP, Eckhouse S. (1996) Photothermal sclerosis of leg veins. *Dermatol Surg* **22**: 323–330.

15. Schroeter CA, Wilder D, Reineke T, *et al.* (1997) Clinical significance of an intense pulsed light source on leg telangiectasias of up to 1mm diameter. *Eur J Dermatol* **7**: 38–42.
16. Fodor L, Ramon Y, Fodor A, *et al.* (2006) A side-by-side prospective study of intense pulsed light and Nd-Yag laser treatment for vascular lesions. *Ann Plast Surg* **56**: 164–170.
17. Sadick NS. (2002) A dual wavelength approach for laser/intense pulse light source treatment of lower extremity veins. *J Am Acad Dermatol* **46**: 66–72.
18. Schroeter CA, Haaf-von Below S, Neumann HA. (2005) Effective treatment of rosacea using the intense pulse light systems. *Dermatol Surg* **31**: 1285–1289.
19. Papageorgiou P, Clayton W, Norwood S, *et al.* (2008) Treatment of rosacea with intense pulse light: significant improvement and long-lasting results. *Br J Dermatol* **159**: 628–632.
20. Neuhaus IM, Zane LT, Tope WD. (2009) Comparative efficacy of nonpurpuragenic pulsed dye laser and intense pulsed light for erythemato telangiectatic rosacea. *Dermatol Surg* **35**: 920–928.
21. Ho WS, Ying SY, Chan PC, *et al.* (2004) Treatment of port wine stains with intense pulse light: a prospective study. *Dermatol Surg* **30**: 887–890.
22. Raulin C, Schroeter CA, Weiss RA, *et al.* (1999) Treatment of port-wine stains with a noncoherent pulsed light source: a retrospective study. *Arch Dermatol* **135**: 679–683.
23. Bjerring P, Christiansen K, Troilius A. (2003) Intense pulse light source for the treatment of dye laser resistant port-wine stains. *J Cosmet Laser Ther* **3**: 7–13.
24. Ozdemir M, Engin B, Mevlitoglu I. (2008) Treatment of facial port-sine stains with the intense pulsed light: a prospective study. *J Cosmet Dermatol* **7**: 127–131.
25. Faurschou A, Togsverd-Bo K, Zachariae C, *et al.* (2009) Pulsed dye laser vs intense pulse light for port-wine stains: a randomised side-by-side trial with blinded response evaluation. *Br J Dermatol* **160**: 359–364.
26. Babilas P, Schreml S, Szeimies RM, *et al.* (2010) Intense Pulsed Light (IPL): A Review. *Lasers Surg Med* **42**: 93–104.
27. McGill DJ, MacLaren W, Mackay IR. (2008) A direct comparison of pulsed dye laser, alexandrite, KTP and Nd-YAG lasers and IPL in patients with previously treated capillary malformations. *Lasers Surg Med* **40**: 390–398.
28. Weiss RA, Goldman MP, Weiss MA. (2000) Treatment of poikiloderma of Civatte with an intense pulsed light source. *Dermatol Surg* **26**: 823–828.
29. Goldman MP, Weiss RA. (2001) Treatment of poikiloderma of Civatte on the neck with an intense pulsed light. *Plast Reconstr Surg* **107**: 1376–1381.
30. Negishi K, Wakamatsu S, Kushikata N, *et al.* (2002) Full-face photorejuvenation of photodamaged skin by intense pulsed light with integrated contact cooling: initial experience in Asian patients. *Lasers Surg Med* **30**: 298–305.
31. Bitter PH Jr. (2000) Noninvasive photorejuvenation of photodamaged skin using serial, full-face intense pulsed-light treatments. *Dermatol Surg* **26**: 835–843.
32. Feng Y, Zhao J, Goldman MH. (2008) Skin rejuvenation in Asian skin: the analysis of clinical effects and basic mechanisms of intense pulsed light. *J Drugs Dermatol* **7**: 273–279.
33. Li YH, Wu Y, Chen JZ, *et al.* (2008) Application of a new intense pulsed light device in the treatment of photodamaged skin in Asian patients. *Dermatol Surg* **34**: 1459–1464.
34. Bjerring P, Christiansen K, Troilius A, *et al.* (2004) Facial photorejuvenation using two different intense pulsed light (IPL) wavelength bands. *Lasers Surg Med* **34**: 120–126.
35. Jorgensen GF, Hedelund L, Haedersdal M. (2008) Long pulsed dye laser versus intense pulsed light for photodamaged skin: a randomised split-face trial with blinded response evaluation. *Lasers Surg Med* **40**: 293–299.
36. Kono T, Groff WF, Sakurai H, *et al.* (2007) Comparison study of intense pulsed light versus a long pulse pulsed dye laser in the treatment of facial skin rejuvenation. *Ann Plast Surg* **59**: 479–483.
37. Cameron H, Ibbotson SH, Dawe RS, *et al.* (2008) Within patient right-left blinded comparision of diode (810nm) laser therapy and intense pulsed light therapy for hair removal. *Lasers Med Sci* **23**: 393–397.
38. McGill DJ, Hutchison C, McKenzie E, *et al.* (2007) A randomised, split-face comparison of facial hair removal with the alexandrite laser and intense pulsed light system. *Lasers Surg Med* **39**: 767–772.
39. Toosi P, Sadighha A, Shaarifian A, *et al.* (2006) A comparison study of the efficacy and side-effects of different light sources in hair removal. *Lasers Med Sci* **21**: 1–4.
40. Amin SP, Goldberg DJ. (2006) Clinical comparison of four hair removal lasers and light sources. *J Cosmet Laser Ther* **8**: 65–68.
41 Bjerring P, Cramers M, Egekvist H, *et al.* (2000) Hair reduction using a new intense pulsed light irradiator and a normal mode ruby laser. *J Cutan Laser Ther* **2**: 63–71.
42. Willey A, Torrontegui J, Azpiazu J, *et al.* (2007) Hair stimulation following laser and intense pulsed light photo-epilation

Review of 543 cases and ways to manage it. *Lasers Surg Med* **39**: 297–301.

43. Radmanesh M, Azar-Beig M, Abtahian A, *et al.* (2008) Burning, paradoxical hypertrichosis, leukotrichia and folliculitis are four major complications of intense pulsed light hair removal therapy. *J Dermatol Treat* **19**: 360–363.
44. Radmanesh M. (2009) Paradoxical hypertrichosis and terminal hair change after intense pulsed light hair removal therapy. *J Dermatol Treat* **20**: 52–54.
45. Chang SE, Ahn SJ, Rhee DY, *et al.* (2007) Treatment of facial acne papules and pustules in Korean patients using an intense pulsed light device equipped with a 530 to 750nm filter. *Dermatol Surg* **33**: 676–679.
46. Yeung CK, Shek SY, Bjerring P, *et al.* (2007) A comparative study of intense pulsed light alone and its combination with photodynamic therapy for the treatment of facial acne in Asian skin. *Lasers Surg Med* **39**: 1–6.
47. Pang AL, Wells K. (2008) Bilateral anterior uveitis after intense pulse light therapy for pigmented eyelid lesions. *Dermatol Surg* **34**: 1276–1279.

Chapter 12

Photodynamic Therapy in the Asian Skin

Colin Thiam-Seng Theng*

Introduction

In 1900, Professor von Tappeiner and his medical student Oscar Raab from the University of Munich, Germany, observed that acridine orange and light killed Paramecium.[1] Three years later, Albert Jesionek and von Tappeiner treated patients with skin tuberculosis and skin cancer with eosin and light, with good results, and the term "photodynamic therapy" was coined.

For the photodynamic reaction to occur, 3 key factors — light, oxygen, and a photosensitizer — must be present.[2] The photosensitizer accumulates in the target tissue and, in the presence of light and oxygen, generates reactive oxygen species resulting in damage and destruction of the target cells.

Photosensitizers

The first-generation photosensitizers were administered systemically. In 1975, hematoporphyrin derivatives were used to treat cancers in animal studies. They are now used for the treatment of a variety of skin cancers and other cancers, including esophageal and bladder carcinomas. Examples of hematoporphyrins include hematoporphyrin derivatives and Photofrin-II (porfimer sodium). The problem with the first-generation photosensitizers was that patients became photosensitive for many weeks as a result of the slow clearance of the photosensitizers from the skin.[3]

The second-generation photosensitizers include the porphines and phthalocyanins. These are similarly systemically administered and, although the clearance is faster than the hematoporphyrins, patients still remain sensitive to sunlight for a period of time. Some of these photosensitizers are activated by light at a longer wavelength and this is useful for the treatment of deeper tumors.

It was with the advent of topical photosensitizers in 1990 that the use of photodynamic therapy (PDT) in dermatology really took off.[4] Topical photosensitizers like 5-amino-levulinic acid (5-ALA) and methyl-aminolevulinic acid (Methyl-ALA) are the main topical preparations used in PDT. Application of these topical photosensitizers lead to localized photosensitivity at the site of application and they are quickly cleared from the skin following treatment. They are prodrugs and are not in themselves photosensitizers. They are taken up by the cells and converted by a series of enzymatic reactions to protoporphyrin IX (PpIX), a photosensitizer within the cell. Most of the photosensitizers are cleared by the heme cycle within 24–48 hours.

Currently, methyl-ALA (Metvix®, Galderma) is approved in Europe, Australia, and the United States for the treatment of actinic keratosis, superficial basal cell carcinoma, and Bowen's disease,[5] together with the use of a red-light source (Aktilite™ 630 nm, Galderma). 5-Aminolevulinic acid (Levulan Kerastick®, Dusa Pharmaceutical) is FDA-approved

*Consultant Dermatologist, Chief, Psoriasis and Phototherapy Unit, National Skin Centre, Singapore.

for the treatment of actinic keratoses in the United States and this is used together with a blue-light source, Blu-U™.[6]

Amino-levulinic acid (ALA) is a small but hydrophilic molecule and is unstable at physiological PH. It is mostly used in concentrations of 20% ALA with incubation periods from 1–18 hours. Being hydrophilic, the tissue penetration of ALA through the lipid bilayer of the stratum corneum may be diminished. Removal of the overlying scales and crusting enhance tissue penetration of the drug. The Levulan kerastick® is used for the treatment of nonhyperkeratotic actinic keratoses and consists of 20% ALA in an alcohol-water solution.

Methyl aminolevulinate (MAL)-PDT is more lipophilic compared with ALA and this allows better penetration of the lipid barrier and cell wall.[7] MAL-PDT is generally regarded to cause less pain compared with ALA-PDT.

Light Sources

Porphyrins have their absorption peak at 410 nm. However, there are smaller peaks at 505, 540, 580, and 630 nm.[8] The amount of activation of the porphyrins depends on the amount of absorption of the light. An activating light in the 410 nm range will be better absorbed by the photosensitizer compared with a light source at 630 nm. However, the shorter the wavelength, the shorter is the depth of penetration into the skin. For activating light sources with lower absorptions, the duration of exposure can be increased to ensure that all the photosensitizers are activated.

Many different light sources have been employed. These include lasers, incandescent filament lamps, and light-emitting diodes (LED). When selecting the light sources, it is important to determine the type of lesion that is being treated. Longer wavelengths (e.g. red light) are preferred for treating skin tumors because of their greater depth of penetration compared with those of a shorter wavelength.

Blue light, 417 nm, has a depth of penetration of about 1–2 mm compared to red light, which has greater depth of penetration (about 6 mm).

Lasers have monochromatic fixed wavelengths and emits radiation at a high intensity. Therefore the duration of treatment is shorter and the side effects of pain and redness are expected to be less. An example of a laser used is the pulsed dye laser (585–595 nm).[9]

Intense pulsed light (IPL) has been used as a light source for facial rejuvenation, treatment of actinic keratoses, and acne.[10]

Incandescent lamps have a wider spectral wavelength output and are safe and easy to use. Examples include the Waldman PDT 1200™.

LED lamps have a medium bandwidth, are relatively less costly, easy to use, and have a large field of irradiation. The LED lamps now have higher photon densities and those currently in use for PDT have higher outputs. Examples include the 630 nm Aktilite 128™.[11]

Recently, ambulatory PDT devices have been developed, where PDT can be delivered by attaching an ambulatory light source on the patient. This decreases the need for the patient to travel to the hospital for treatment.[12,13] There have been a number of reports of the use of ambient light for PDT.[14,15] This was employed for the treatment of actinic keratoses and the slow, continuous activation of the photosensitizers decreases the pain of treatment, with reported good efficacy.

There are also reports of the benefit of fractionation of the light exposure to improve the clinical response to PDT. Fractionation allows for improved oxygen delivery during periods when the oxygen supply may be exhausted and thus enhances the photodynamic response.[16]

The protocols for PDT are varied, e.g. for LED light sources, the usual doses used range from 37 to 75 J/cm^2 and for other broadband lamps, the doses range from 75 to 150 J/cm^2.

Indications for Photodynamic Therapy

Major Indications	Promising Indications	Reported to be Effective
Actinic keratosis	Actinic cheilitis	Darier's disease
Bowen's disease	Cutaneous T cell lymphoma	Disseminated superficial actinic porokeratosis
Superficial basal cell carcinoma	Viral warts	Hailey-Hailey disease
Nodular basal cell carcinoma	Lichen sclerosus	Nercobiosis lipoidica
	Field Cancerisation	Epidermodysplasia verruciformis
	Photorejuvenation	Psoriasis
		Sarcoidosis
		Extramammary Paget's Disease
		Nephrogenic fibrosing dermopathy
		Mycobacterium marinum
		Erythrasma
		Rosacea

Mechanism of Action

ALA is a prodrug and not a photosensitizer. It is a precursor in the heme synthesis pathway and is converted by a series of enzymes to protoprophyrin IX (PpIX), which is the photosensitizer.[4] In the heme synthesis pathway, there are 2 key rate-limiting enzymes — ALA synthase and ferrochelatase. ALA synthase produces ALA from glycine and succinyl CoA. When ALA is applied in large amounts topically, this is absorbed by the cell and there is accumulation of the ALA within the cell. This bypasses the first rate-limiting enzyme, ALA synthase. After ALA is absorbed in the cell, it is rapidly converted via the enzymatic pathway to PpIX. As ferrochelatase is the second rate-limiting enzyme, PpIX accumulates in the cell, as it is produced at a much faster rate than can be cleared by the cell. This results in a localized porphyria-like state in the cell. Sufficient time has to be given to enable the ALA to penetrate the cell and be metabolized to produce an adequate concentration of PpIX, which peaks after 3–15 hours of ALA application.

In tumor cells, there is a preferential uptake of the ALA into the tumor. The epidermis overlying the diseased area is often damaged, and this allows for better penetration of the ALA. Furthermore, tumor cells have reduced ferrochelatase activity, due to a relative lack of ferric ions in the cells, leading to even more accumulation of the PpIX.[16]

The optimal duration of incubation may vary. Different incubation times from 1–48 hours have been used in different protocols. The ideal incubation time varies according to the underlying pathology. In general, there is a trend toward shorter incubation times for nonmalignant indications such as facial rejuvenation and acne vulgaris.

When the protoporphyrin is activated by the light, reactive oxygen species is generated. This results in destruction of the cells by direct damage and by induction of apoptosis. The reactive oxygen species

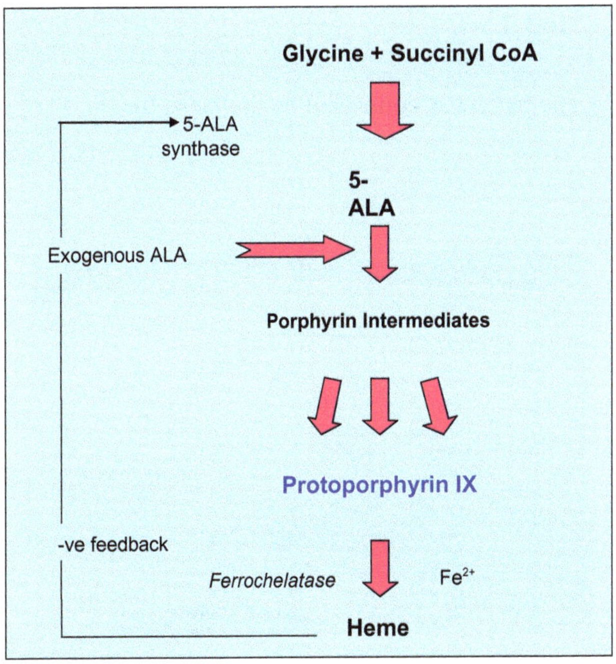

The enzymatic pathway in heme synthesis. Exogenous ALA bypasses the first rate-limiting enzyme, ALA synthase.

has a very short half-life of <1 nanosecond (ns), and the primary targets are the mitochondria, lysosomes, and plasma membrane.[17] As it does not appear to result in damage to DNA, the number of treatments can be repeated as necessary and the risk of carcinogenesis from repeated treatments appears to be very remote.

The PDT Treatment

A variety of PDT protocols have been used that vary in the incubation times, ranging from 1–16 hours. In general, the incubation time for ALA is 4–6 hours and the incubation time for MAL is 3 hours, which is the protocol with the use of the Aktilite 128™ or Aktilite 16™ LED lamp. The Aktilite is preset to deliver 37 J/cm^2 and the machine automatically shuts down when the dose is delivered.

The following outline the steps in performing photodynamic therapy with MAL-PDT.

Step 1

The patient is counseled on the steps for the PDT.

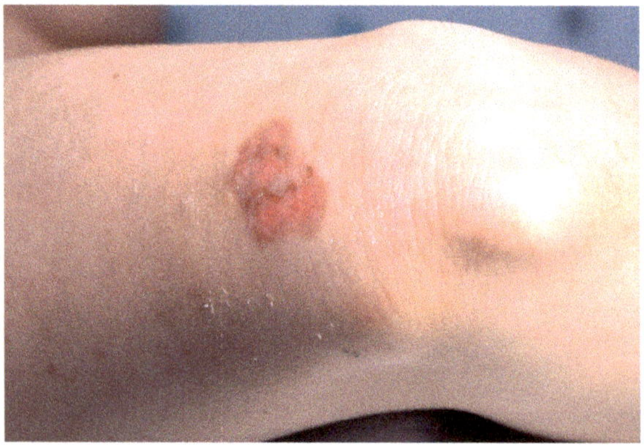

Step 2

After the lesion is identified, the overlying scales and crusts are removed to allow for better penetration of the cream. Any areas of oozing are compressed firmly to arrest the bleeding.

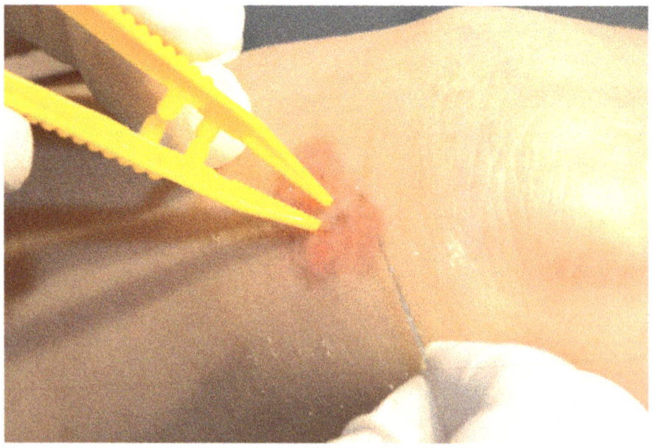

Step 3

Topical MAL is then applied evenly to the area. This is at least 1–2 mm thick and extends 5–10 mm beyond the border of the lesion, which corresponds to a "surgical margin" around the lesion.

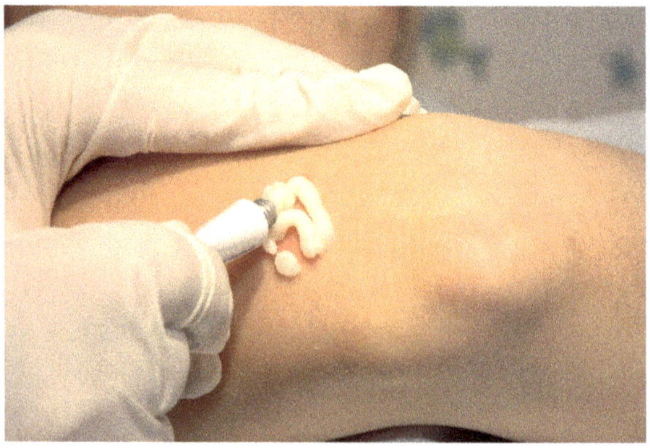

Step 4

The area is occluded with a dressing such as Tegaderm®.

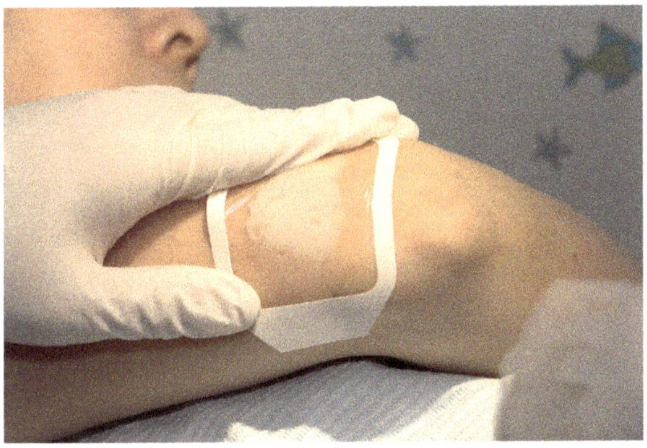

Step 5

An opaque dressing is applied over the lesion to prevent the photosensitizer from being activated by the ambient light and is left on for the duration of the incubation period, which is three hours with MAL.

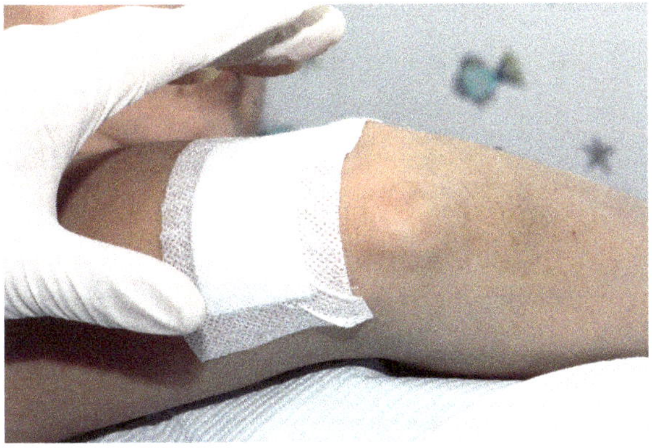

Step 6

After three hours of occlusion, the dressing is removed, the cream is wiped off, and the area cleansed with normal saline.

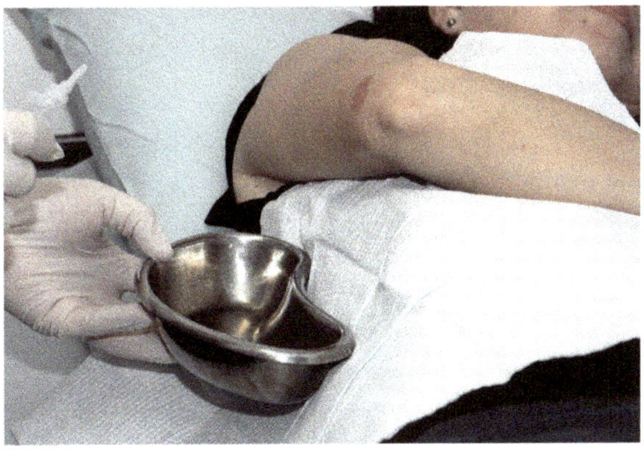

Step 7

The Aktilite™ LED red light is positioned over the area at a distance of 5–8 cm away from the lesion. During the irradiation, cold-water sprays may be used to reduce the discomfort. The duration of the irradiation is 7–10 min.

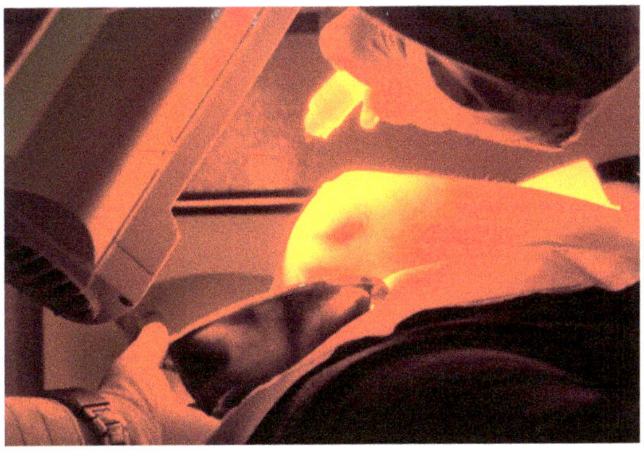

Postprocedure Care

Immediately post treatment, the pain and discomfort diminishes once the light irradiation ceases, but the patient may experience discomfort that can linger for 24 hours or more. A cold compress to the treatment area can be given to relieve the discomfort, and oral analgesics like paracetamol may be taken.

The treated area may blister and ooze for a few days, followed by inflammation and crusting for a few days. The crust will peel off after about 7–10 days. Normal saline may be given to cleanse the area and white soft paraffin may be applied. An opaque dressing may be applied over the lesion and the patient is advised to avoid sun exposure for the next 24–48 h.

Side Effects of PDT

Photodynamic therapy is a phototoxic event and therefore the anticipated side effect is a phototoxic reaction on the skin. Pain is often felt during the procedure and is described as tingling and burning. The degree of pain varies from minimal discomfort to severe pain. The pain typically starts during irradiation of the light, gradually increasing. It peaks after a few minutes and rapidly diminishes on discontinuation of the irradiation. Erythema and swelling usually occurs and, occasionally, an urticarial response can be seen at the irradiation site.[18]

Although it is difficult to accurately predict who will develop severe pain from the treatment, the following may help to identify the patient with a higher risk of developing PDT pain:

1. Extent of the lesion — the larger the area, the greater the pain
2. Site of the lesion — the face, scalp and genital areas are more painful
3. Type of lesion — treatment for actinic keratosis is more painful than for basal cell carcinoma
4. Type of treatment — ALA-PDT is generally more painful than MAL-PDT.

Commonly used methods for pain relief include fanning or spraying cold water over the treated area. Cold-air analgesia has also been used. EMLA® cream or tetracaine gel has been shown to be no better than placebo in modulating the pain.[19] Other methods to decrease the pain include the use of transelectric nerve stimulation[20] and fractionated PDT, where the irradiation treatment is interrupted.

Local anesthesia (without adrenaline) can be used in cases where the pain is severe. However, it can be difficult to administer to large areas. More recently, there have been reports of the effective use of nerve blocks, such as supraorbital and occipital nerve blocks, to decrease the pain when treating extensive actinic keratoses on the face and scalp.[21] This has become routine practice in some European centers.

Other side effects include post-inflammatory hyperpigmentation (PIH). This problem is particularly common in Asian patients and patients with darker skin types.[22] This usually resolves in 3–6 months. Other reported side effects include hair loss, which can be permanent.

The risk of carcinogenicity with repeated treatments of PDT appears to be low, but more long-term follow-up studies are needed to confirm this.

Photodynamic Therapy for Actinic Keratoses

Actinic keratosis is a precancerous lesion, characterized by dysplastic epidermal keratinocytes. It is caused by damage of the skin from cumulative sun exposure and occurs commonly on the scalp, face, and extensors of the forearms. Due to the increased risk of transformation to squamous cell carcinoma, actinic keratoses should be treated.

Treatment modalities include cryotherapy and topicals such as imiquimod, 5-fluorouracil (5-FU) and diclofenac sodium. PDT has been used to treat actinic keratoses with good clinical results.

In the United States, 20% ALA in the form of an alcohol-water solution, Levulan Keratick® with blue light is FDA-approved for the treatment of actinic keratoses.[23,24] ALA is applied 14–18 h over the actinic keratoses before the blue light irradiation is carried out. No occlusion is necessary. The main side effects are pain during the irradiation and erythema after the treatment. This is more pronounced when a larger area is being treated at one sitting.

In Europe, methyl-ALA PDT is more commonly employed for the treatment of actinic keratoses. The incubation period is three hours, followed by irradiation at 37 J/cm^2 with the red light at 632 nm. Initial protocols recommended two treatments, one week apart, and efficacy ranged from 70–100%.[25] A recent study treating 1501 actinic keratoses in 119 patients showed that a single treatment with MAL PDT followed by a repeat treatment at three months had equally effective outcomes compared with two PDT treatments one week apart. The clearance was reported at 92% and 87% respectively.[26] The current recommendation is a single treatment repeated at three months, if necessary.

Actinic keratoses respond better to PDT if the lesions are thin. Those on the scalp and face fare better than those on the forearms.

In Asians, there is an increased risk of PIH following PDT treatment, which may limit its use in treating larger areas of photodamaged skin or actinic keratoses.

Case 1: An 81-year-old Chinese man had a history of squamous cell carcinoma of the left thigh and Bowen's disease that had been excised. He presented with scattered, scaly erythematous papules on the forehead consistent with actinic keratoses (Fig. 12.1). He underwent a single MAL-PDT treatment.

Case 2: A 78-year-old Chinese man had multiple actinic keratoses on the right cheek that were treated with single session of PDT, with excellent improvement (Fig. 12.2).

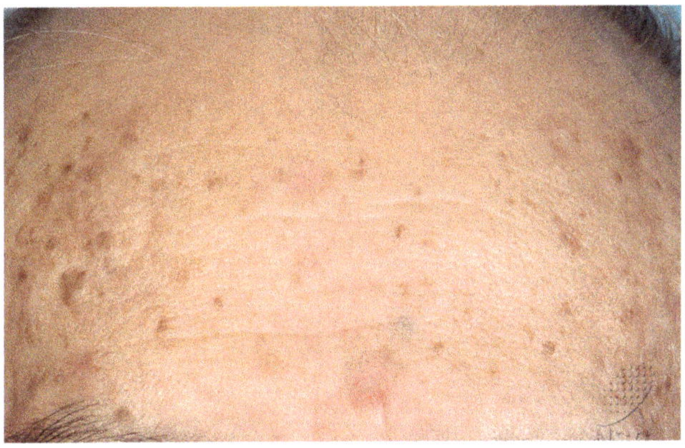

Pretreatment: Actinic keratoses on the forehead.

3 months post-treatment with a single session of Methyl-ALA PDT.

Figure. 12.1.

Actinic keratoses.

Photodynamic Therapy for Bowen's Disease

Bowen's disease, or squamous cell carcinoma-in-situ, has a 3–5% risk of transformation to invasive squamous cell carcinoma. It is common on sun-exposed sites but can occur in covered areas, e.g. the genitals.

Treatment options for Bowen's disease include surgical excision, curettage and electrosurgery, cryotherapy, and topicals, e.g. 5-fluorouracil and imiquimod. PDT is an effective option, with reported clearance rates of 86–93% following 1–2 treatments.[5]

A multicenter randomized controlled study comparing MAL-PDT with 5-FU and cryotherapy was carried out on 225 patients, with 275 lesions treated.[27]

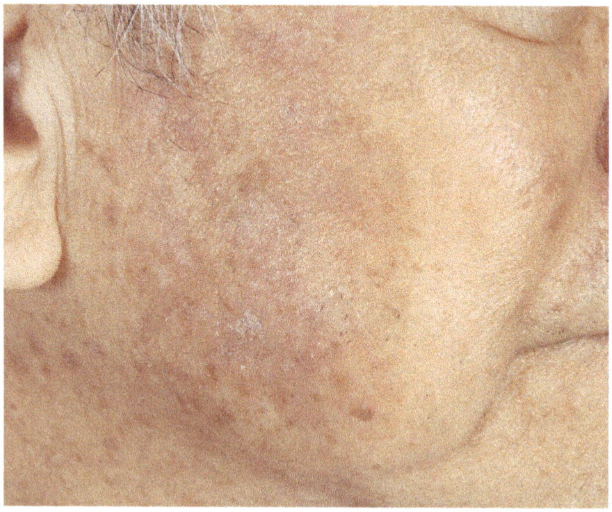

Pretreatment: Actinic keratoses on the right cheek.

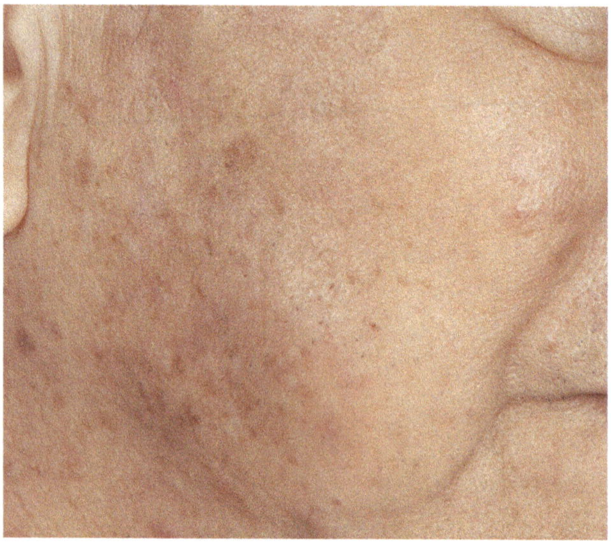

1 month following a single session of Methyl-ALA PDT.

Figure. 12.2.

Actinic keratoses.

At three months, the clearance rate of Methyl-ALA PDT, cryotherapy, and 5-FU was 86%, 82%, and 83% respectively. At the 24-month follow-up, the clearance rate was 68%, 60%, and 59% respectively. Superior cosmetic outcome was noted in the PDT-treated group.

Photodynamic therapy for Bowen's disease is particularly useful for sites with poor wound healing, such as the lower legs in elderly patients and in patients with multiple lesions. There have been reports of the use of PDT in unusual sites such as the nipple, subungual, and eyelid areas.[28–30]

The guidelines for the treatment of Bowen's disease is one cycle of two PDT treatments, spaced one week apart. The patients are evaluated at three months and treated again if necessary.

We have treated patients with skin type IV with MAL-PDT and have noted excellent results. Recurrence rates, however, are higher, especially in patients who are immunosuppressed.

In our Asian context, arsenic ingestion from traditional Chinese medications leading to arsenical keratoses and multiple Bowen's disease have responded well to PDT treatment, an ideal option in this group of patients, as multiple sites can be treated simultaneously and the lesions heal very well.

It is important to have a pretreatment biopsy to confirm the diagnosis of Bowen's disease. If multiple treatments have been given and the lesion does not clear, it should be re-biopsied to rule out invasive squamous cell carcinoma.

In summary, PDT is an appropriate treatment for Bowen's disease, with good clearance rates and an excellent cosmetic outcome.

Case 3: An 87-year-old Chinese man was referred with biopsy-confirmed Bowen's disease on his right thigh. He underwent 2 Methyl-ALA PDT treatments, at one week apart, with complete clearance of the Bowen's disease and excellent healing post PDT (Fig. 12.3).

Case 4: A 47-year-old man presented with a persistent scaly rash on the penile shaft for over a year. A skin biopsy confirmed Bowen's disease. He received two treatments of Methyl-ALA PDT, at 2 weeks apart. His lesion had clinically resolved at the 3-month follow-up (Fig. 12.4). Unfortunately, a recurrent papule was noted at the 6-month follow-up and he elected for electrocautery.

Case 5: A 67-year-old Chinese man presented with a large scaly patch that had been on the left wrist for years. Biopsy confirmed Bowen's disease. He declined surgery and was treated with two treatments of MAL

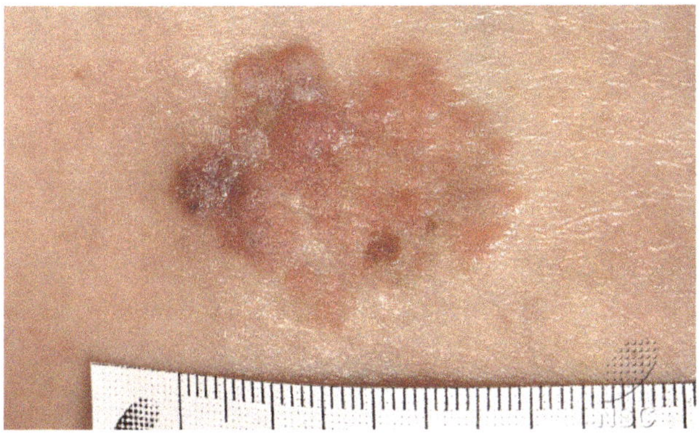

Pretreatment: Bowen's disease on the right thigh.

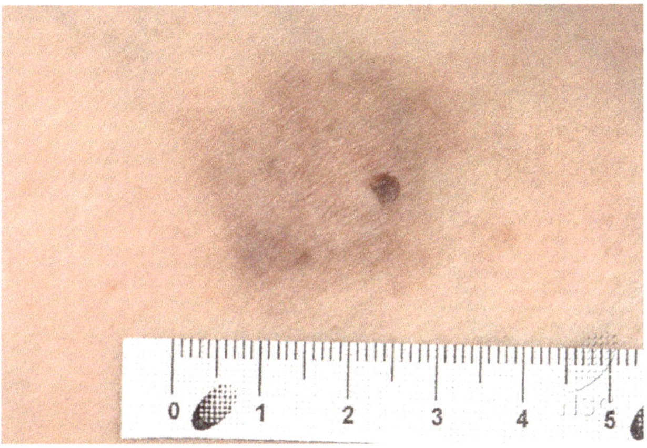

3 months post-treatment with 2 MAL-PDT sessions 1 week apart .

Figure 12.3.

Bowen's disease.

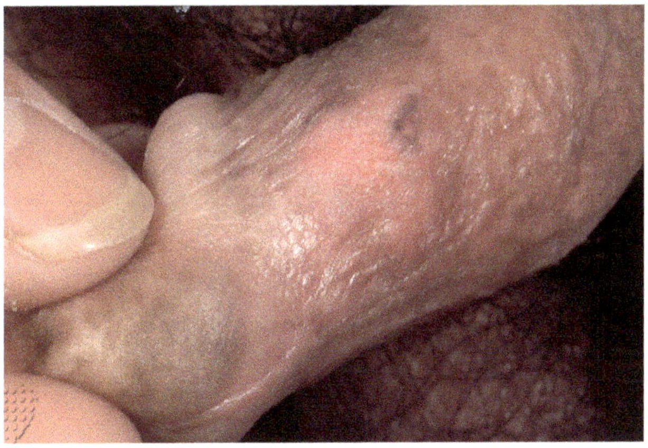

Pretreatment : Bowen's disease on the penile shaft.

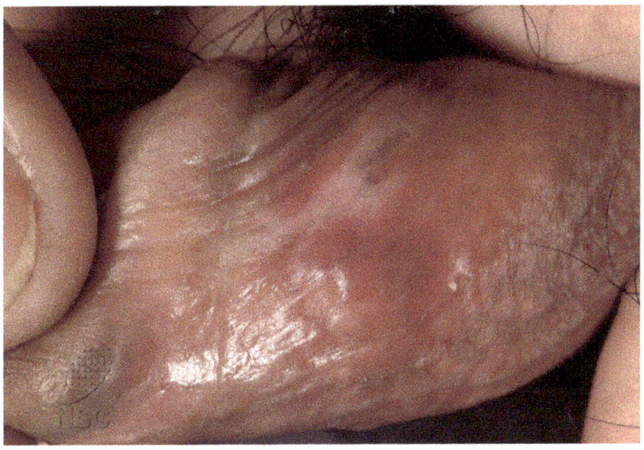

Bowen's disease 3 months post-treatment with 2 sessions of Methyl-ALA PDT, two weeks apart.

Figure 12.4.

Bowen's disease.

PDT, at one week apart (Fig. 12.5). The Bowen's disease had completely cleared at the 3-month follow-up and he remains clinically clear at two years post treatment.

Photodynamic Therapy for Basal Cell Carcinoma

PDT is licensed in Europe for the treatment of superficial and nodular basal cell carcinomas (BCC).

Numerous studies had demonstrated the effectiveness of PDT in BCC: efficacy ranged from 82–100% for superficial BCC.[5,25]

Primary superficial basal cell carcinomas that are < 1 cm outside the H zone area of the face are considered good prognostic factors.[31]

The main advantage of PDT over surgery is its better cosmetic outcome.

Initial studies on PDT for nodular BCC showed reduced efficacy.[5] For nodular BCC, prior debulking curettage improves the outcome. One study reported that, with debulking curettage for nodular BCC prior to PDT, a clearance of 92% was achieved.[32] Rhodes *et al.* reported that, for small nodular BCCs treated with MAL-PDT (two treatments one week apart), clearance rate at three months was 91%, vs 98% with surgery.[33] The 12-mth response rate was 83%, vs 96%

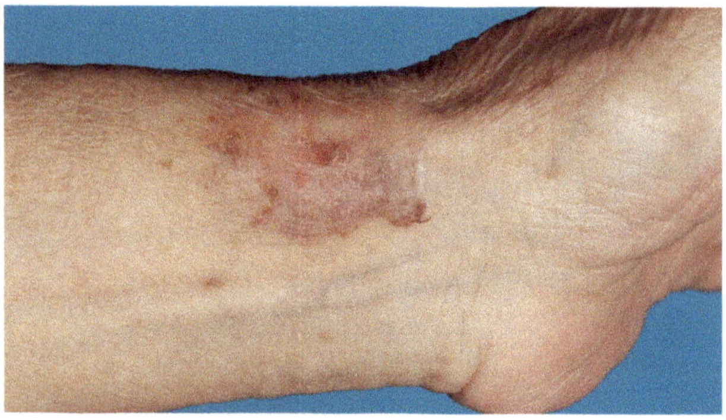

Pretreatment: Bowen's disease on the right wrist.

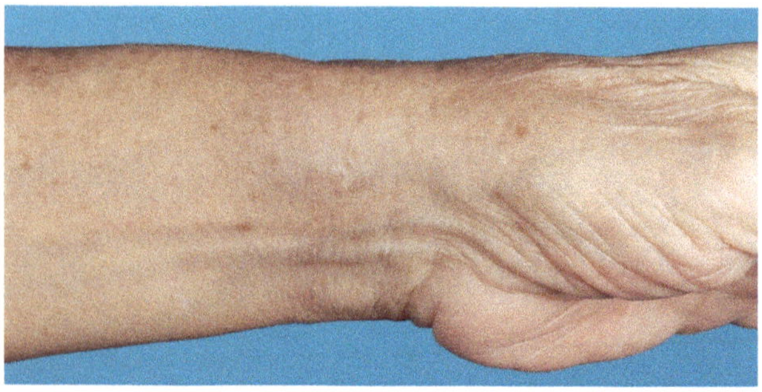

3 months post-treatment with 2 Methyl-ALA PDT sessions one week apart.

Figure 12.5.

Bowen's disease.

with surgery. At the 5-year follow-up, the sustained response rate for surgery was 96%, compared with 76% for MAL-PDT.[34]

In Asian skin, the pigmented variant of BCC is more commonly encountered. Pigmented BCC responds less well to PDT treatment with lower clearance and higher recurrence rates. PDT is not indicated for morpheic basal cell carcinoma.[5]

Case 6: A 96-year-old Chinese woman presented with a growth just below her right eyebrow area for a month. Biopsy confirmed a superficial basal cell carcinoma. She received two treatments of Methyl-ALA PDT, at one week apart (Fig. 12.6). The lesion cleared and remained clear on review a year later.

Case 7: An 89-year-old Chinese woman had a 2-year history of a growth on the nose that was slowly enlarging. Biopsy confirmed a micronodular basal cell carcinoma. She received two treatments of Methyl-ALA

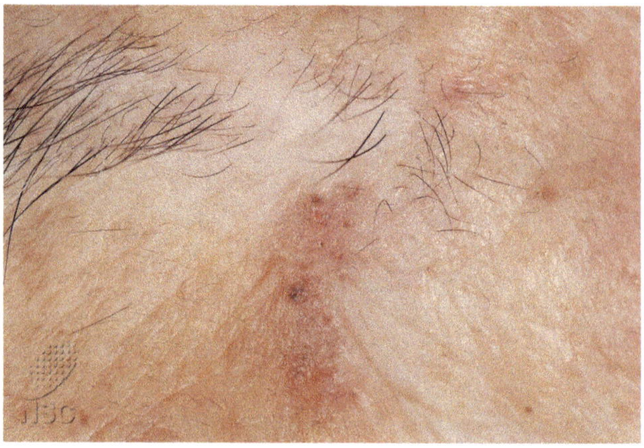

Pretreatment: Superficial BCC below the right eyebrow area.

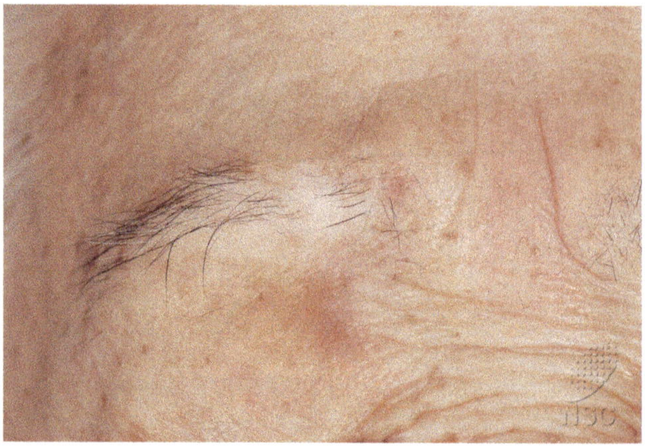

1 month post-treatment with 2 MAL-PDT sessions a week apart.

Figure 12.6.

Basel cell carcinoma.

PDT at one week apart and had clearance of the lesion at the 3-month follow-up (Fig. 12.7).

Photodynamic Therapy for Cutaneous T Cell Lymphoma

Cutaneous T cell lymphoma (CTCL) is an uncommon group of conditions, with the most common being T cell and NK cell forms. They present in the early stage with patch- and plaque-stage mycosis fungoides (MF), and in the later stages with tumor-stage MF.

The largest series to date has treated 10 patients with 12 lesions of MF with PDT and the number of treatments, ranged from 2 to 11.[35] Seven of the lesions completely responded but none of the tumor-stage lesions responded to treatment.

There are other reports on the improvement of mycosis fungoides with PDT.[36,37] At present, there is no standardized protocol for the treatment of MF.

In the management of cutaneous T cell lymphoma, PDT has a possible role in the treatment of limited or isolated CTCL, particularly in patch- and plaque-stage MF.

Case 8: A 14-year-old Chinese girl was diagnosed with localized mycosis fungoides, confirmed on histology. She had received multiple treatments with phototherapy and radiotherapy but the plaque persisted. She received eight sessions of PDT at 1–3 weekly intervals (Fig. 12.8). There was thinning of the plaque post PDT and a repeat biopsy showed no evidence of MF. She is currently on follow-up.

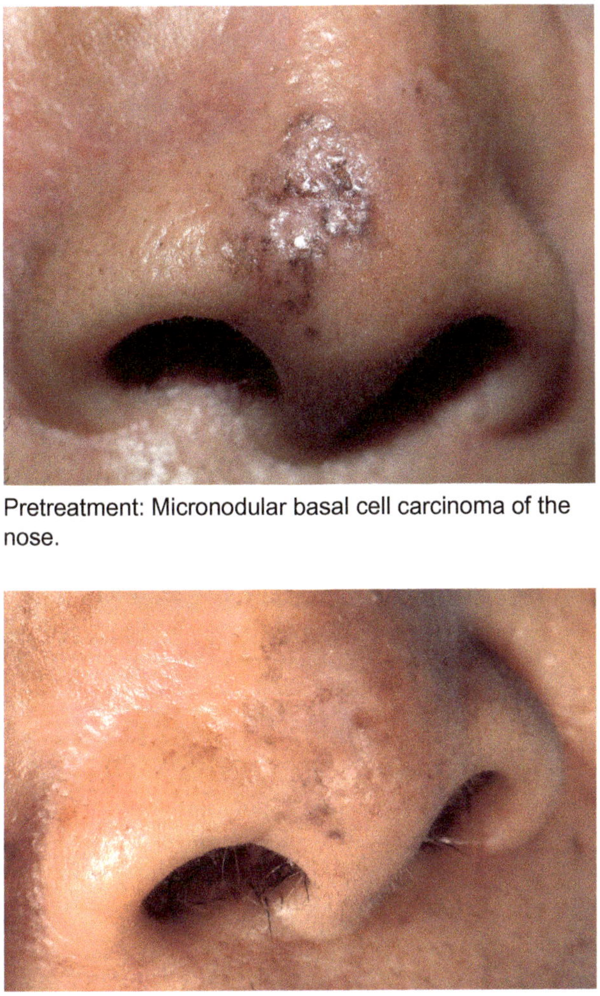

Pretreatment: Micronodular basal cell carcinoma of the nose.

Three months post-treatment with 2 MAL-PDT treatments, 1 week apart.

Figure 12.7.

Basel cell carcinoma.

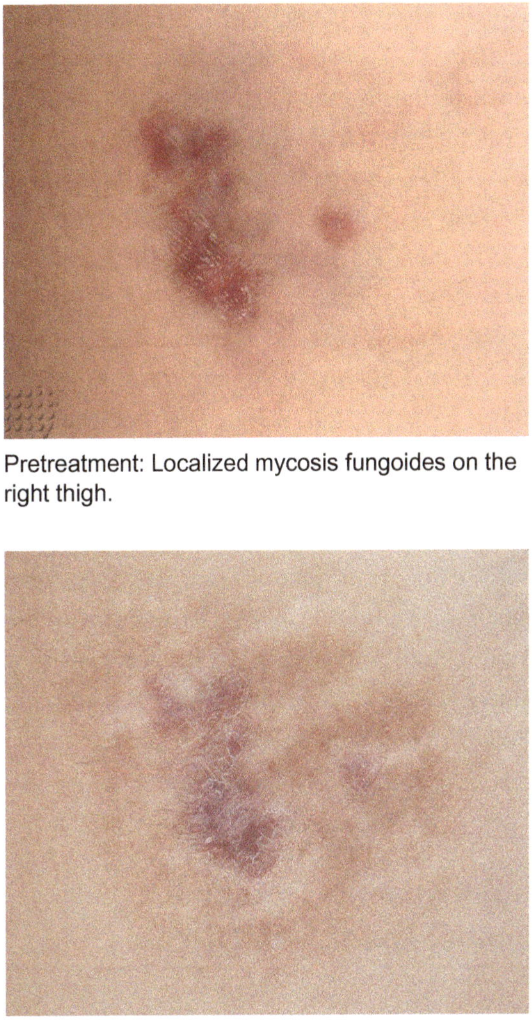

Pretreatment: Localized mycosis fungoides on the right thigh.

Post-treatment: After multiple sessions of Methyl-ALA PDT, spaced at 1- to 3-weekly intervals, flattening of the plaque was achieved.

Figure 12.8.

Mycosis fungoides.

Photodynamic Therapy for Extramammary Paget's Disease

There are reports on the efficacy of PDT for the treatment of extramammary Paget's disease (EMPD). A report from Japan, of two patients with histologically proven EMPD treated with PDT using 5-ALA, showed clearance at three months, following two sessions of PDT.[38] The second case also cleared after 3 PDT sessions but recurrence was noted at the margins. However, this cleared with 2 further treatment sessions.

A review of five patients with 16 EMPD lesions, treated with ALA-PDT and red light, showed clearance in 8 of the lesions after six months. However, three lesions recurred after 3–4 months.[39]

Topical PDT can be a potentially effective treatment of EMPD. However, recurrence of the disease is likely to be high and surgery remains the treatment of choice in these patients.

Case 9: An 82-year-old Chinese man presented with a one-year history of an itchy rash on the genital area. Examination showed an erythematous plaque on the scrotum and penis. A biopsy confirmed extramammary Paget's disease. He was referred for PDT of the EMPD, as surgery was contraindicated in view of his history of lung disease. He received two treatments of Methyl-ALA PDT a week apart, with good clinical clearance (Fig. 12.9). A repeat biopsy showed histological clearance. However, the lesion recurred 10 months later.

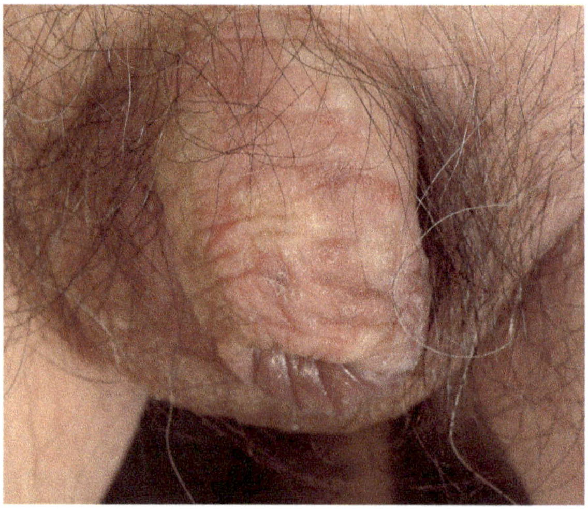

Pretreatment: Extramammary Paget's disease affecting the shaft of the penis.

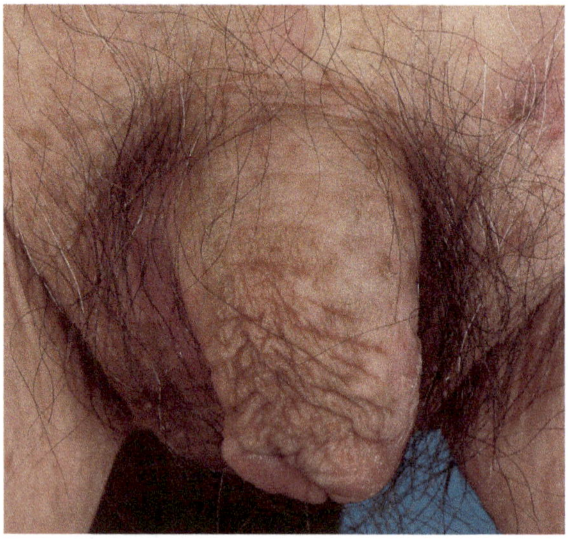

Three months post-treatment of extramammary Paget's disease, showing good clinical improvement.

Figure 12.9.

Extramammary Paget's disease.

Photodynamic Therapy for Nonmalignant Skin Diseases

PDT for Acne Vulgaris

In recent years, there has been increasing interest in the use of light-based therapy for acne vulgaris. PDT provides an alternative to antibiotic-based therapy and may be useful in cases where antibiotic therapy has failed and where patients do not wish to be on oral antibiotics for prolonged periods. With the increasing antibiotic resistance in acne, PDT may become an increasingly viable option.

PDT works in acne vulgaris by targeting *P acnes* that produce endogenous porphyrins. These are activated by irradiation with blue light, resulting in the generation of singlet oxygen, which destroys the bacteria. When ALA is applied, it is taken up by the pilosebaceous units and converted to PpIX. Irradiation with light then results in apoptosis and damage to the sebaceous glands, leading to a decrease in sebum production.[40]

In Asian skin, one of the key concerns is the development of PIH, which can limit the use of PDT in the treatment of acne vulgaris.

There are no standard protocols on the use of PDT for acne vulgaris. Photosensitizers such as 5-ALA and methyl ALA have been used to treat acne. There is a trend toward shorter incubation and irradiation times in the treatment of benign conditions. Light sources that have been used include blue light, red light, PDL, and IPL.

A review of published data on PDT and acne vulgaris suggested that topical short-contact (90 min or less) 5-ALA or Methyl-ALA, using a noncoherent light source at 2–4 week intervals for 2–4 treatments, produces good clinical improvement.[41] Papulopustular lesions responded better to the treatment and skin types I–III have lower risk of PIH, which is seen more commonly in darker skin.

A study of 78 Chinese patients with grade 4 severe acne vulgaris treated with topical 5-ALA PDT was recently published.[42] Forty-two patients were treated with 1–3 courses: 10% ALA cream was applied topically to the acne lesions for 3 hours, followed by irradiation with an LED light of 633 nm at doses of 50–70 J/cm^2 at 66 mW/cm^2. After a single course of treatment, 22% of patients showed excellent improvement and 34% showed excellent improvement after two sessions. The remainder (44%) required three sessions to further reduce the number and size of residual lesions. Minimal adverse events were observed.

In a split-face treatment from Thailand involving 14 patients with acne vulgaris, one side was treated with short-contact topical ALA and IPL and the other side with IPL alone. The decrease in lesion count was 87.7% at 12 weeks on the ALA-treated side and 66.8% on the IPL-treated side. Mild edema and minimal crusting were noticed on the ALA-IPL-treated sides.[43]

In our experience, we have found that a single treatment of either 5% or 20% ALA, incubated for three hours and irradiated with red light, resulted in an improvement of the inflammatory acne and comedone count in truncal acne (Figs. 12.10, 12.11). This improvement may be seen within the first two weeks, although a small proportion of patients may have an initial flare during the first two weeks. The main problem is the development of PIH (Fig. 12.12). In our initial series of 17 patients with skin type IV–V, most patients developed mild hyperpigmentation, but one patient developed severe PIH. The PIH resolved in all patients within 3–6 months.

Case 10

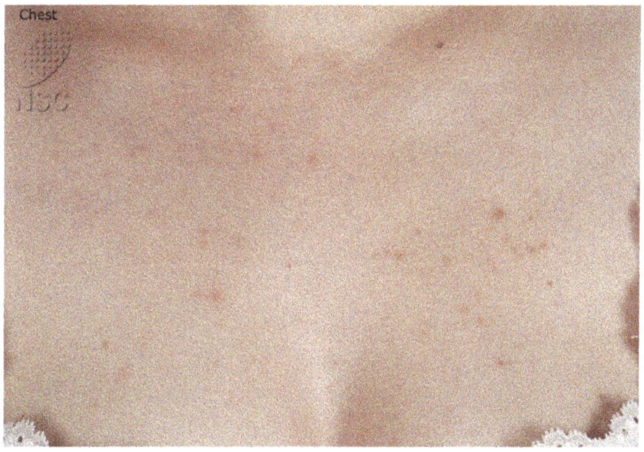

Pretreatment: Acne on the chest.

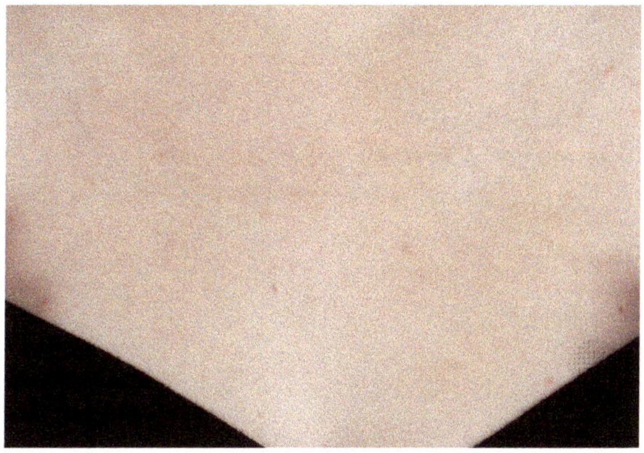

Three months post-treatment after a single treatment of 5% ALA PDT, showing marked improvement in the inflammatory papule count.

Figure 12.10.

Acne vulgaris.

Case 11

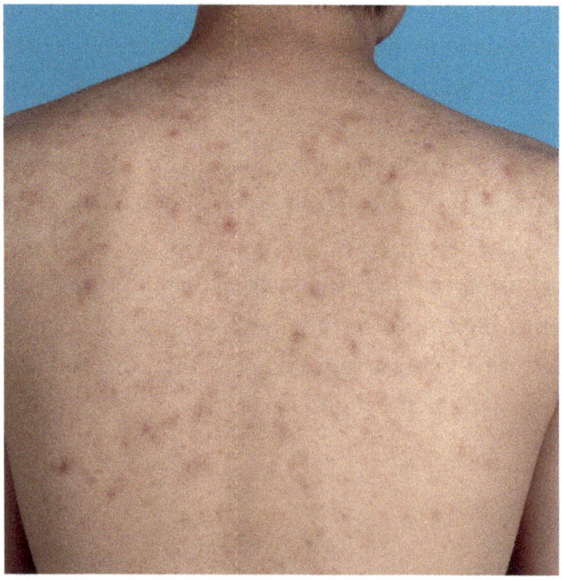

Pretreatment: Truncal acne on the back.

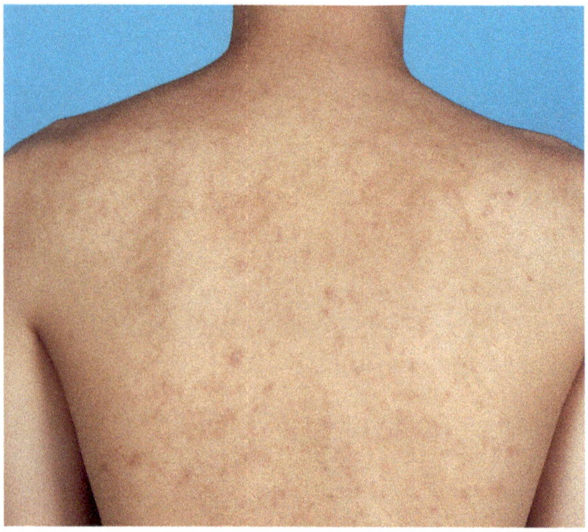

Three months post-treatment after a single treatment of 5% ALA PDT showing good improvement in the acne.

Figure 12.11.

Acne vulgaris.

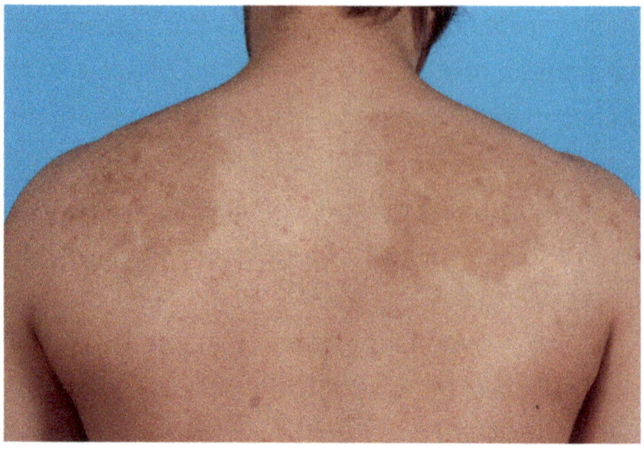

Marked post-inflammatory hyperpigmentation at 1 month post 20% ALA PDT treatment for truncal acne, which resolved completely in 6 months.

Figure 12.12.

Post-inflammatory hyperpigmentation.

PDT for Viral Warts

There have been numerous studies on the use of PDT for the treatment of viral warts, with reported clearance rates ranging from 56–100%.[25]

A prospective, single-arm study of 5-ALA PDT in the treatment of recalcitrant viral warts in an Asian population was carried out.[44] Recalcitrant warts were surgically pared, then treated with 20% 5-ALA cream under occlusion for 4 hours before irradiation with a red light source (Waldmann PDT1200; wavelength, 590–700 nm) at an irradiance of 50 mW/cm^2 and a total dose of 50 J/cm^2. Treatment was repeated fortnightly for a maximum of 4 times. Of the 12 patients treated, five patients (42%) showed complete disappearance of the warts, one patient (8%) showed partial clearance (greater than 50% decrease in the wart area), five patients (42%) had stable disease (less than 50% decrease in the wart area), and one (8%) showed progressive disease. Treatment was generally well tolerated.

We reported a 20-year-old man who presented with a 3-month history of a recalcitrant viral wart on the right thumb, which failed numerous weekly cryotherapy sessions.[45] He was treated with three MAL-PDT sessions weekly and his wart cleared completely a month later (Fig. 12.13).

Peri-ungual warts are difficult to treat. A study from Korea examined the combination of ablative CO_2 fractional laser and methyl-ALA PDT for the treatment of recalcitrant periungual warts.[46] Twelve Korean patients with a total of 40 peri-ungual warts were treated with the ablative CO_2 fractional laser, followed immediately by the application of MAL and irradiated with red light three hours later. A mean of 2.2 treatments were carried out and clearance of the lesions was noted in 36 (90%) of the peri-ungual warts. Two warts had 50% clearance, and 2 showed no response after three treatments.

For the treatment of viral warts, PDT can be considered in cases resistant to other forms of treatment. The option of combining with other modalities such as fractional lasers to enhance penetration of the photosensitizer is attractive. However, the routine use of PDT for the treatment of warts is limited by the cost of treatment and unpredictability of the response.

PDT for Other Indications

PDT has been reported to be effective for numerous skin diseases. Most of these are based on case reports or small case series, and additional work is needed before PDT can be incorporated into routine use for their treatment.

Lichen sclerosus has been reported to respond well to treatment with PDT: in particular, itching improves significantly. Other promising indications include the use of PDT in the treatment of cutaneous leishmaniasis and in the treatment of field cancerization. PDT is also a promising modality for photorejuvenation.

Other conditions that have been reported to benefit from PDT treatment include Hailey-Hailey disease, sarcoidosis, epidermodysplasia verruciformis, Darier's disease, lichen planus, nevus sebaceous, sebaceous hyperplasia, rosacea, erythrasma, mycobacterium marinum infection, nephrogenic fibrosing dermopathy, and disseminated superficial actinic porokeratosis.[5,25]

Case 12

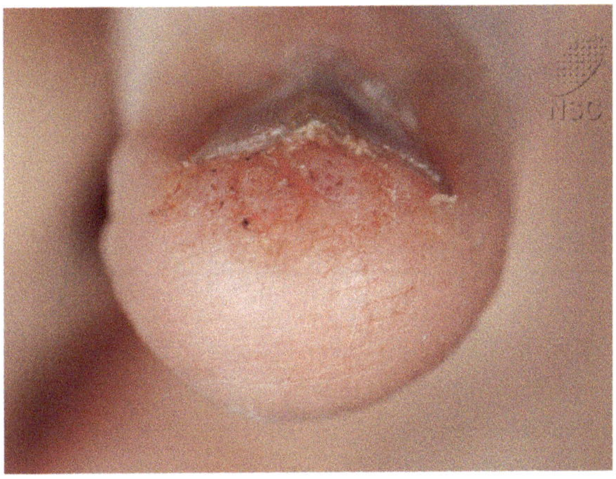

Pretreatment: Persistent periungual wart.

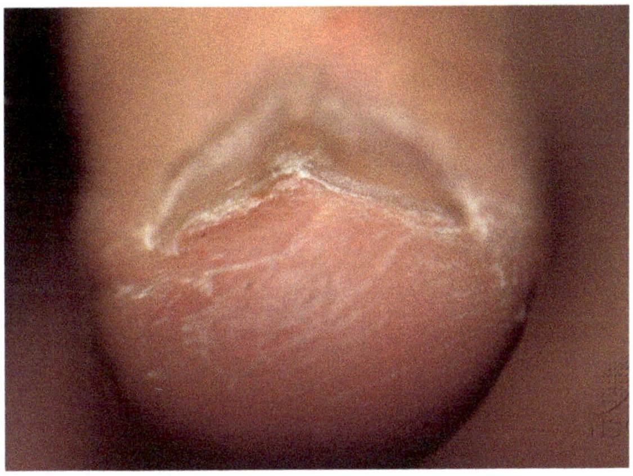

Marked improvement following 3 Methyl-ALA PDT treatments.

Figure 12.13.

Viral wart.

Conclusion

PDT is a simple, noninvasive treatment for many skin conditions, both benign and malignant, with excellent cosmetic outcomes. While it does not replace surgery, it is certainly an attractive option in cosmetically and functionally sensitive sites and on areas of poor wound healing. Its indications will likely increase to include many more skin diseases but more studies and defined protocols need to be developed to determine its optimal delivery. In Asian skin, post-inflammatory hyperpigmentation is significantly higher than in Caucasian skin and care should be taken, especially when treating for cosmetic indications.

References

1. Daniell MD, Hill JS. (1991) A history of photodynamic therapy. *Aust N Z J Surg* **61**: 340–348.
2. Henderson BW, Dougherty TJ. (1992) How does photodynamic therapy work? *Photochem Photobiol* **55**: 145–157.
3. Dougherty TJ, Cooper MT, Mang TS. (1990) Cutaneous phototoxic occurrences in patients receiving photofrin. *Lasers Surg Med* **10**: 485–488.
4. Kennedy JC, Pottier RH, Pross DC. (1990) Photodynamic therapy with endogenous porphyrin IX: basic principles and present clinical experience. *J Photochem Photobiol B Biol* **6**: 143–148.
5. Morton CA, Brown SB, Collins S, *et al.* (2001) Guidelines for topical photodynamic therapy: report of a workgroup, the British Photodermatology Group. *Br J Dermatol* **145**: 75–78.
6. Omrod D, Jarvis B. (2000) Topical aminolevulinic acid HCL photodynamic therapy. *Am J Clin Dermatol* **1**: 133–139.
7. Gersher S, Connelly JP, Beijersbergen van Henegouwen GM, *et al.* (2001) A quantitative assessment of protoporphyrin IX metabolism and phototoxicity in human skin following dose-controlled delivery of prodrugs 5-aminolaevulinic acid and 5-aminolaevulinic acid-n-pentylester. *Br J Dermatol* **144**: 983–990.
8. Pottier RH, Chow YFA, LaPlante JP, *et al.* (1986) Non invasive technique for obtaining fluorescence excitation and emission spectra *in vivo*. *Photochem Photobiol* **44**: 679–687.
9. Karrer S, Baumler W, Abel C, *et al.* (1999) Long-pulse dye laser for photodynamic therapy: investigations *in vitro* and *in vivo*. *Lasers Surg Med* **25**: 51–59.
10. Babilas P, Schreml S, Szeimiers RM, *et al.* (2010) Intense pulse light (IPL): a review. *Lasers Surg Med* **42**: 93–104.
11. Juzeniene A, Juzenas P, Ma LW, *et al.* (2004) Effectiveness of different light sources for 5-aminolevulinic acid photodynamic therapy. *Lasers Med Sci* **19**: 139–149.
12. Moseley H, Allen JW, Ibbotson S, *et al.* (2006) Ambulatory photodynamic therapy: a new concept in delivering photodynamic therapy. *Br J Dermatol* **154**: 747–750.
13. Attili SK, Lesar A, McNeill A, *et al.* (2009) An open pilot study of ambulatory photodynamic therapy using a wearable low-irradiance organic light-emitting diode light source in the treatment of nonmelanoma skin cancer. *Br J Dermatol* **161**: 170–173.
14. Marcus SL, Houlihan A, Lundahl S, *et al.* (2007) Does ambient light contribute to the therapeutic effects of topical photodynamic therapy (PDT) using aminolevulinic acid (ALA)? *Lasers Surg Med* **39**: 201–202.
15. Batechelor RJ, Stables GI, Stringer MR. (2007) Successful treatment of scalp actinic keratoses with photodynamic therapy using ambient light. *Br J Dermatol* **156**: 779–781.
16. Svanberg K, Andersson T, Killander D, *et al.* (1994) Photodynamic therapy of non-melanoma malignant tumours of the skin using topical delta-aminolevulinic acid sensitization and laser irradiation. *Br J Dermatol* **130**: 743–751.
17. Szeimies RM, Karrer S, Abels C, *et al.* (2001) Photodynamic therapy in Dermatology. In: Krutmann J, Honigsmann H, Elmets CA, *et al.* (eds.), *Dermatological Phototherapy and Photodiagnostics Methods*, pp. 209–247. Springer, Berlin.
18. Clark C, Dawe RS, Moseley H, *et al.* (2004) The characteristics of erythema induced by topical 5-aminolevulinic acid photodynamic therapy. *Photodermatol Photoimmunol Photomed* **20**: 105–107.
19. Langan SM, Collins P. (2006) Randomized, double-blind, placebo-controlled prospective study of the efficacy of topical anaesthesia with a eutectic mixture of lignocaine 2.5% and prilocaine 2.5% for topical 5-aminolaevulinic acid-photodynamic therapy for extensive scalp actinic keratoses. *Br J Dermatol* **154**: 146–149.
20. Halldin CB, Paoli J, Sanderg C, *et al.* (2008) Transcutaneous nerve stimulation for pain relief during photodynamic therapy for actinic keratosis. *Acta Derm Venereol* **88**: 311–313.
21. Serra-Guillen C, Hueso L, Nagore E. (2009) Comparative study between cold air analgesia and supraorbital and supratrochlear nerve block for the management of pain during photodynamic therapy for actinic keratoses of the frontotemporal zone. *Br J Dermatol* **161**: 353–356.
22. Chan HH. (2005) Efficacy and safe use of lasers, light sources, and radiofrequency devices in the clinical management of Asian patients with selected dermatoses. *Lasers Surg Med* **37**: 179–185.
23. Rivard J, Ozog D. (2006) Henry Ford Hospital dermatology experience with levulan Kerastick and blue light photodynamic therapy. *J Drugs Dermatol* **5**: 556–561.

24. Lang K, Schulte KW, Ruzicka T, *et al.* (2001) Aminolevulinic acid (Levulan) in photodynamic therapy of actinic keratoses. *Skin Therapy Lett* **6**: 1–2, 5.
25. Morton CA, McKenna KE, Rhodes LE, *et al.* (2008) Guidelines for topical photodynamic therapy: update. *Br J Dermatol* **159**: 1245–1266.
26. Tarstedt M, Rosdahl I, Berne B, *et al.* (2005) A randomized multicenter study to compare two treatment regimens of topical methyl aminolevulinate (Metvix®)-PDT in actinic keratosis of the face and scalp. *Acta Derm Venereol* (Stockh) **85**: 424–428.
27. Morton CA, Horn M Leman J, *et al.* (2006) Comparison of topical methyl aminolevulinate photodynamic therapy with cryotherapy or fluorouracil for treatment of squamous cell carcinoma in situ: results of a multicenter randomized trial. *Arch Dermatol* **142**: 729–735.
28. Brookes PT, Jhawar S, Hinton CP, *et al.* (2005) Bowen's disease of the nipple — a new method of treatment. *Breast* **14**: 65–67.
29. Usmani N, Stables GI, Telfer NR, *et al.* (2005) Subungual Bowen's disease treated by topical aminolevulinic acid photodynamic therapy. *J Am Acad Dermatol* **53**(Suppl. 1), S273–S276.
30. Calista D, Coccia L. (2008) Photodynamic therapy for the treatment of in situ squamous cell carcinoma of the left eyelid. *Int J Dermatol* **47**: 1319–1321.
31. Vinciullo C, Elliot T, Francis D, *et al.* (2005) Photodynamic therapy with topical methyl aminolaevulinic acid for 'difficult to treat' basal cell carcinoma. *Br J Dermatol* **152**: 765–772.
32. Thissen MR, Schroeter CA, Neumann HA. (2000) Photodynamic therapy with delta-aminolaevulinic acid for nodular basal cell carcinomas using a prior debulking technique. *Br J Dermatol* **142**: 338–339.
33. Rhodes LE, de Rie M, Enstrom Y, *et al.* (2004) Photodynamic therapy using topical methyl aminolevulinate vs surgery for nodular basal cell carcinoma: results of a multicenter randomized prospective trial. *Arch Dermatol* **140**: 17–23.
34. Rhodes LE, de Rie MA, Leifsdottir R, *et al.* (2007) Five-year follow-up of a randomized, prospective trial of topical methyl aminolevulinate photodynamic therapy vs surgery for nodular basal cell carcinoma. *Arch Dermatol* **143**: 1131–1136.
35. Edstrom DW, Ros AM. (2001) Photodynamic therapy with topical 5-aminolevulinic acid for mycosis fungoides: clinical and histological reponse. *Acta Derm Venereol* (Stockh) **81**: 184–188.
36. Coors EA, von den Driesch P. (2004) Topical photodynamic therapy for patients with therapy-resistant lesion of cutaneous T-cell lymphoma. *J Am Acad Dermatol* **50**: 363–367.
37. Zane C, Venturini M, Sala R, *et al.* (2006) Photodynamic therapy with methylaminolevulinate as a valuable treatment option for unilesional cutaneous T-cell lymphoma. *Photodermatol Photoimmunol Photomed* **22**: 254–258.
38. Mikasa K, Watanabe D, Kondo C, *et al.* (2005) 5-Aminolevulinic acid-based photodynamic therapy for the treatment of two patients with extramammary Paget's disease. *J Dermatol* **3**: 97–101.
39. Shieh S, Dee AS, Cheney RT, *et al.* (2002) Photodynamic therapy for the treatment of extramammary Paget's disease. *Br J Dermatol* **146**: 1000–1005.
40. Hongcharu W, Taylor CR, Chang Y, *et al.* (2000) Topical ALA-photodynamic therapy for the treatment of acne vulgaris. *J Invest Dermatol* **115**: 183–192.
41. Taylor MN, Gonzalez ML. (2009) The practicalities of photodynamic therapy in acne vulgaris. *Br J Dermatol* **160**: 1140–1148.
42. Wang XL, Wang HW, Zhang LL, *et al.* (2010) Topical ALA PDT for the treatment of severe acne vulgaris. *Photodiagnosis Photodyn Ther* **7**: 33–38.
43. Rojanamtin J, Choawawanich P. (2006) Treatment of inflammatory acne vulgaris with intense pulse light and short contact of topical 5-aminolevulinic acid: a pilot study. *Dermatol Surg* **32**: 991–996.
44. Wang YS, Tay YK, Kwok C, *et al.* (2007) Photodynamic therapy with 20% aminolevulinic acid for the treatment of recalcitrant viral warts in an Asian population. *Int J Dermatol* **46**: 1180–1184.
45. Chong WS, Kang GY. (2009) Dramatic clearance of a recalcitrant acral viral wart using methyl aminolevulinate-red light photodynamic therapy. *Photodermatol Photoimmunol Photomed* **25**: 225–226.
46. Yoo KH, Kim BJ, Kim MN. (2009) Enhanced efficacy of photodynamic therapy with methyl 5-aminolevulinic acid in recalcitrant periungual warts after ablative carbon dioxide fractional laser: a pilot study. *Dermatol Surg* **35**: 1927–1932.

Index

www.ingramcontent.com/pod-product-compliance
Ingram Content Group UK Ltd.
Pitfield, Milton Keynes, MK11 3LW, UK
UKHW051045150926
8624IPUK00006B/406